"As Ava's pediatric oncologist, I discussed with her and her family the "four legs of the stool" that we would use to guide her cancer journey. The first three are traditional medical tools-chemotherapy, surgery and radiation, and the fourth equally important leg is hope. In *From Cancer to Kinnick: Love Finds a Wave*, Jeff offers a glimpse into this intimate part of their cancer journey and how faith and hope gave them the crucial strength of resilience. This story of Ava, Jeff and their amazing family is inspiring and sheds light on the importance that faith in something bigger than ourselves; can bring us strength and hope in the most difficult of times. *From Cancer to Kinnick: Love Finds a Wave* provides an intimate and inspiring narrative of the cancer journey. Jeff provides an inspiring account of how faith and hope are crucial in the most difficult times."
—**William W. Terry, MD, MPH, Medical Oncologist, Clinical Associate Professor, Co-Director of the Adolescent and Young Adult Cancer Program, UIHC**

"In my 5 years as Principal at Jordan Catholic School, Ava Hoskins has shown her strength, faith, and determination to continue to get healthier. Watching Ava continually push through all of the adversity has been an inspiration to all of her peers and staff that have watched her grow over the years. Ava demonstrates a confidence that is unparalleled, and has the biggest heart for others. She is growing into a young woman who will continue to do wonderful things for others, because her amazing family has led by example!"
—**Mr. Jacob A. Smithers, Principal, Jordan Catholic School**

FROM CANCER TO KINNICK
Love Finds A Wave

Jeff Hoskins
with Ava Hoskins

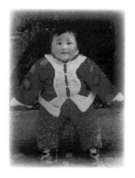

Ice Cube Press, LLC
North Liberty, Iowa, USA

From Cancer to Kinnick: Love Finds A Wave

Copyright ©2021 Jeff Hoskins

First Edition

Isbn 9781948509251

Library of Congress Control Number: On file

Ice Cube Press, LLC (Est. 1991)
1180 Hauer Drive
North Liberty, Iowa 52317 USA
www.icecubepress.com | steve@icecubepress.com

The paper used in this publication meets the minimum
requirements of the American National Standard
for Information Sciences—Permanence of Paper for
Printed Library Materials, ANSI Z39.48-1992.

Manufactured in USA using recycled paper.

Author proceeds from the sale of this book will be
donated to the Stead Family Children's Hospital.

TO

Ava, a gentle warrior and my hero
Brady and Macy, the best siblings a little girl could have
Renae, the love of my life
Drs. William Terry & Jamie Truscott, for saving my daughter
Kinnick Wavers, for giving love and hope

AND

Ad majorem Dei gloriam

Although the world is full of suffering, it is also full of the overcoming of it.
—Helen Keller

Contents

Introduction

by Ava Hoskins

*Appreciation is a wonderful thing. It makes what is
excellent in others belong to us as well.*
—Voltaire

Hello, my name is Ava Hoskins. I first want to thank you for
reading this book. I hope that you will be inspired. During my
journey through cancer I have learned lots of things. Cancer
changed my perspective on life. If I could go back and change the
past, of course I wouldn't want cancer, but I am thankful for who
I am because of it. I am a living miracle of God and I'm proud
that I get this opportunity to inspire and help others. I love the
saying "expect the unexpected." When I first learned I had cancer,
I expected it to be horrible and my life would never be the same
again. It turned out that there are many good things that came
along the journey too. You sometimes just have to look a little
harder. I also learned that it was true, life would never be the same
again, but I could still enjoy it.

I would have never been able to do this without my family and
friends. During my journey I was very lucky to have both my sister and brother at the University of Iowa. They visited me all the
time. We would eat lunch together and hang out. I felt more safe
and comfortable knowing my brother and sister were nearby. My
parents worked their butts off! They had to juggle so much, yet
they got through it with a positive attitude. They did everything

they could do to make sure I was ok. I missed a lot of school because I was either neutropenic, tired, didn't feel well, or I was at the hospital. I was lucky to have teachers that understood and helped me while dealing with cancer. They allowed me to work at my own pace so that I could learn too. Along with that, I have amazing friends who supported me. I am forever grateful to them, the doctors and other hospital staff, and everybody else who has helped me through this unexpected journey.

My Hope

The sun shone warm and bright on August 2nd, 2016. As it set that evening, we had no idea by the time we saw it again the next morning our lives would be forever changed. This book begins with the odyssey to adopt our youngest daughter, Ava, and ends with our battle to save her life, beginning that fateful evening.

This is not a medical manual, a managing cancer how-to guide, or a what-to-expect when you're side-effecting compendium. What it is, is an honest and heartfelt look at having a child with cancer, how that led to an outpouring of love towards our family, and a reminder that good can be found even when you least expect it. The purpose of this book is fourfold:

1. To give thanks.
2. To give hope.
3. To inspire the giving of love and hope.
4. To show love, peace, joy and beauty can be present even in the worst of circumstances.

I want to give thanks to God for providing strength and peace to our family and for placing so many beautiful people in our life to help us carry the cross of a critically ill child. I'd like to give hope to those who may be similarly struggling, and even to those that aren't. The world can seem so loveless and hopeless at times, but we can attest it is still very much filled with both love and hope and, therefore, with God.

I also hope this book inspires people to give love and hope.

As you'll see in these pages, love can come in many different forms, from Slurpees to waving to dancing, but it always involves generosity. Generosity is love in action, and hopefully this book encourages the giving of one's time, talent, and treasure to those in need around them. One's love is a currency of infinite and eternal value, but only when it is spent on others. Finally, I hope this book shows that love and peace and joy and beauty can be found even in the worst of circumstances. Helplessly watching your child suffer is undeniably painful. But like salve on a wound, love given by others can bring a joy, peace, and beauty that helps ease that pain.

I was watching a presentation by a priest recently and he wrote on the whiteboard, "God never gives me more than I can handle." He asked the group if we had heard that phrase before and everyone agreed. Then, surprisingly, he said he completely disagreed. He went on to say God quite often gives each of us more than can be handled on our own. The more correct wording, he explained, is really, "God never gives me more than *we* can handle." What God gives us is meant to be gone through not just by ourselves, but united to Him and with our family, friends, neighbors, and community. As he said this I immediately thought how my family is living proof of that. Suffering is supposed to be a group project, and we had a wonderful group help us through ours.

I used to watch those St. Jude commercials on television and my heart would go out to the parents as they told their stories. I could not imagine what it would be like to have a child with cancer or any other potentially fatal illness. I always prayed for them, then thanked God it was not our family. I believed there was no way we would be able to survive such an ordeal. I literally would die. Then I blinked, and our daughter Ava was one of those kids, and we were one of those families. I was right, we could not have survived our daughter's cancer diagnosis on our own. However, by the grace of God and the love and prayers of many people, we survived. This book is a glimpse into our experience of hope and love during the trying, and not so trying, times.

Before the Beginning

If you want to make God laugh, tell him your plans.
—St. Teresa of Calcutta

We should have seen it coming. Ava gave us an entire year after she was born to prepare, then she cannon-balled into our family, took over, ... and made our lives joyfully complete.

My wife Renae and I wrongly thought our family was complete long before Ava was born. In 1995 we entered the world of parenthood with the birth of our daughter Macy, and then completed Parenthood: The Sequel when our son Brady was born in 1996. Two kids. One boy. One girl. A complete set. No one ever has to sit by themselves on a roller coaster. We were done!

God laughed.

Over the next few years Renae and I kicked around the idea of adopting a child. We thought God was calling us to adopt a child from the foster care system so in 2001 we took a sixteen week Illinois Foster Parenting course and became licensed foster parents. It wasn't long before we realized the process was not going to be for us. We only wanted to foster children available for adoption, but that did not happen. And, in spite of our training, we felt unable to give these kids the support they needed. Finally, we knew people who had attempted to adopt this way who ended up having children removed from their home when a relative of the child came forward. All of this was way more than we were prepared to handle so we figured God didn't know what he was talking about and we put an end to our thoughts of adopting. We were going to remain a family of four and keep our seat mates on the roller coaster.

God laughed a little harder.

Renae and I met at Illinois State University in the Fall of 1987. We were both pursuing Bachelors of Science degrees in Environmental Health. Eventually we started dating and in October of 1992 we were married. I tell our kids fate brought us together, but Renae swears alcohol must have been involved somehow. We lived in the Chicago area after college as well as during our first couple of years of marriage. I worked in downtown Chicago and Renae worked in the suburbs. In 1994 we received the wonderful news that we were expecting our first child! With that life-changing news came a life-changing decision. We decided we wanted Renae to be a stay-at-home mom. There was a minor flaw in our plan however. We felt there was no way we could survive in Chicago on my meager income. After much discussion, we left the area of Renae's childhood, Chicago, and moved to the area of my childhood, the Quad Cities. Rock Island, Illinois to be exact. With great self-sacrificing love Renae gave up her career and familiar surroundings to move, in her words, "to the sticks."

We felt God gave us a thumbs up we were doing the right thing when soon after we made the decision I landed a job in the Quad Cities doing exactly what I did in Chicago and I was even going to make a little more money! That was the first time I realized God was involved and will always give us what we need in order to do what he wants us to do.

Fast forward a few years. Since Macy and Brady were in school and the adoption-through-foster-parenting thing fell through,

Renae decided she wanted to go back to school to become a nurse. So, in 2003 she became a student again.

In nursing school, one thing that annoyed Renae to no end were assignments that had nothing to do with nursing, such as the time she gave a presentation on adolescents in Amish communities. She saw the exercises as a complete waste of time. She would have much rather spent the time learning things like, say, how to take care of sick people.

In the Spring of 2004 Renae's class was assigned to give a presentation on an aspect of a foreign culture. Once she recovered from her head exploding, she got to work on her presentation. And by saying "she" got to work I mean "we" got to work. Renae has a great many talents but technology is not one of them, so whenever she had a project due she became project manager and I became both research assistant and technical support. Providentially, the topic she chose for this particular assignment was China's one-child policy. This controversial policy was initiated to control China's population growth by restricting the number of children a family could have. The policy resulted in hundreds of thousands of children, mostly girls, either being aborted or abandoned. As we sat together at the computer researching this program, a collective lightbulb went off above our heads and in our hearts. We knew then, with absolute certainty, what our calling was—to adopt a daughter from China. I guess her assignment wasn't so meaningless after all.

That summer we researched international adoption agencies and officially started our adoption journey by applying at a local agency in October, 2004. The next several months were spent gathering entire forests of paperwork, documenting everything from what our childhood was like to how well the local police department "knew" us. Finally, on December 16, 2005, our plethora of paperwork arrived at the China Center of Adoption Affairs (CCAA) in Beijing. When we started the process, the waiting period between the arrival of a couple's paperwork in China and the arrival of a referral from China (introducing our new child) was only six months, so we fully expected to bring our new baby home by the summer of 2006. We were a little bummed because this meant we might have to miss Renae's nursing school graduation.

Again, God laughed…really, really hard.

Almost the Beginning[1]

The waiting is the hardest part.
—Tom Petty

I'll never forget the brutal morning of January 24, 2008. The dashboard clock read 6:30AM, and the deep, black night seemed uninterested in conceding its icy grip. The darkness only magnified the glowing temperature display as it shouted 18 degrees *below* zero. It was going to be a long day. This was the scene as Renae and I began our third trip in as many years to be fingerprinted again at the US Citizenship and Immigration Services office in Naperville, Illinois, one of the many requirements for adopting a child from China.

Despite the fact that fingerprints are as permanent as a Chicago Cub fan's loyalty, the Department of Homeland Security declares them expired fifteen months after being printed. Just to be sporting, before our trip I called the department for an explanation of this rule. I eventually spoke with an actual human who clarified it quite succinctly: "Umm . . . I don't know why. That's just the policy." Well, there it was. I felt much better about traveling three hours to spend another $200 to confirm our fingerprints hadn't changed.

Due mainly to the increased number of people wanting to adopt from China and CCAA not increasing the number of children available for adoption, we developed a serious case of "wait"

---

1 Reprinted and adapted with permission from *Celebrate Life* Magazine.

gain as our expected six short months had grown into a tough twenty-four.

During this excruciating time, in addition to our fingerprinting trifecta, we also had to renew our formal request to bring an orphan into this country. I looked up the word "renew" in the dictionary and learned it's a French word meaning "to write a large check." And that we also had to do again. We not only felt as if we were throwing money down the drain but we literally had to put our adoption money into the sewer, thanks to the untimely demise of the sewer line in front of our house during this time. And we had to reproduce several other documents since they had expired. Our troubles included one that was notarized with a stamp that didn't have a box around it, rendering both the stamp and document invalid. Boxless stamps must be what terrorists use when they notarize.

Finally, on January 3, 2008, we received our referral, complete with photos and information about our daughter! But our excitement was tinged with anxiety, since we had to wait another six weeks to meet her, as well as finalize plans for a sixteen-hour flight and required two-week stay in China. On this final trip to Naperville, I remember reflecting on all we had invested in this adoption process, from the money to the time spent compiling paperwork, to the agonizing wait, to the tedious hoops we had to jump through. However, I also remember thinking that I already loved this child so much I would do it all again and there was nothing I wouldn't do to have her with me. It was then, in the cold and quiet of that morning I could sense God saying, "And now you know what My love is like."

The Beginning—Finally!

*Not flesh of my flesh, nor bone of my bone, but still
miraculously my own. Never forget for a single minute,
you didn't grow under my heart, but in it.*
—Fleur Conkling Heyliger

Prior to adopting Ava I never had any interest in traveling to China. Europe, yes. South America, maybe. But China? That just seemed too...international. I was pleasantly surprised how much I enjoyed it once we were there though. Getting to China was an adventure all its own. It started at the Quad City International Airport in Moline, Illinois, after we had checked ourselves and our luggage in. We cleared security and were sitting in the concourse about an hour before our flight was to leave. Thankfully Brady noticed on the flight screen that instead of our flight leaving at 9:31AM it now read "Now departing at 11:30AM." This was a big problem since our connecting flight from Chicago to China was leaving at 12:17PM. We were able to get a flight on American Airlines that left at 10:30AM, which cut our connection very close but was doable. Since it was so close, the computer system at American would not register our luggage. The agents had to hand write tags for our bags which, in my mind, guaranteed them to be lost. We did make it to Chicago in the nick of time and, after running from one end of O'Hare Airport to the other like the family in the *Home Alone* movie, we got to our connecting terminal just as they were starting to board.

The flight was v-e-r-y long and uneventful. Adoption is not for the faint of heart, and neither is international air travel. At one point I dozed off and when I woke up I figured we must be almost there. To my dismay I had only slept twenty minutes and there were still six hours to go. I thought it was interesting our flight didn't actually travel from East to West but more North to South. We flew up through Canada to just south of the North Pole and then came down through Siberia. Every once in a while they flashed the temperature on the television screen. It read "-79° F" for a very long time.

The good news was we made it safely to China. The bad news was our luggage did not. Well, three of our five pieces didn't. However, considering we expected none of our luggage would make it we were pleasantly surprised.

We spent our first two days in Hong Kong before leaving to get Ava. It's a beautiful city. It was like a clean and friendly Chicago. Everywhere we looked someone was cleaning something. The people were extremely friendly and very helpful. There were people in every mall, hotel, park, etc. standing around waiting to help tourists find what they needed or to get them where they wanted to go. The weather was in the sixties and most everything was green. Even the flowers were in bloom. This was awesome since we knew at home it was snowing and the temperature in the 20's. Most everyone in Hong Kong spoke English in addition to Chinese, and all of the signs were in both English and Chinese. Curiously, most of the advertisements used Caucasian models. One thing that struck me was the number of children I saw in the area. Almost as many as there were Starbucks.

After our two days in Hong Kong we flew about 575 miles north to the city of Wuhan. Yes, that Wuhan, future epicenter of the

COVID outbreak. My first impression was...*this ain't Hong Kong*. I was reminded that we were now in a communist country when, instead of the smiling faces and brightly dressed agents as in the Hong Kong airport, we were greeted by somber military style uniforms with faces to match. As soon as we got through the check-in booth with our passports it was a shift change for the agents. We watched as they all lined up single file and marched in unison into another room.

We will never forget the bus ride from the airport to our hotel. The driving in China was completely insane. There were usually at least two vehicles, a moped and a dozen pedestrians jockeying for the same lane at any given time. We had our eyes closed most of the way. I kissed the ground when we got to our hotel.

Unlike Hong Kong, virtually no one in Wuhan spoke English, and none of the signs were in English. It was quite an eerie feeling. What was also eerie, but hilarious too, was when we took a walk to a grocery store to get some supplies. You would have thought we had green skin, purple hair, and horns growing from our heads. Everyone stared at us. Apparently they don't get many gringos in those parts.

The next day was "Gotcha Day"—the day we finally got Ava. The day started with another exciting bus ride, this time to the Office of Civil Affairs of the Hubei Province, the province where Wuhan is located. When we arrived we were told to have our cameras ready because once we were in the building, things were going to happen very fast. Including us, there were ten other families receiving their child that day. We were part of the first group to arrive. We walked in and sat down at a large table, and in the corner was a woman holding a baby—the only one in the room. One of the Civil Affairs workers started speaking and then our guide came over to tell us that was Ava! The director of her orphanage was holding her and playing with her, and we had to sit there waiting for this lady to finish jabbering and then sign a bunch of papers! We were so close.

We have no idea what we signed. We could have joined the military for all we know. We just wanted to get Ava. Finally, in this drab conference room in the middle of this city I'd never heard of on the other side of the world, I was able to hold my beautiful new daughter. As I gazed at her I learned a lesson I will never forget: You can't outgive God!

It was so incredible to finally hold her! There were no words to describe having her in my arms. The whole event took place in less than an hour. One minute we left the hotel as a family of four, a few minutes later we returned as a family of five.

The next morning we returned to the Office of Civil Affairs to finalize the adoption (as far as China was concerned). It went pretty quick. A few signatures, fingerprints (again!), a short interview, bada boom bada bing and she was ours! As we left the building and waited to board the bus, a couple of elderly women happened to be walking by and came up to us. They started speaking Chinese, of course. The thing I learned about the Chinese language is you can't tell if people are carrying on a normal conversation or if they're wishing a thousand deaths upon you and your ancestors. Anyway, these ladies were smiling and giving us a thumbs up. One of the ladies then started crying. We turned to our interpreter wondering what was going on. She said the ladies were very touched that we would come to their country to adopt these abandoned children. As we pulled away one of the older women was wiping away her tears and gave us another thumbs up.

Afterwards we went to a mall to pick up some more things, including clothes for Renae since most of hers were in San Francisco and who knows where else. The mall was very modern and sold just about everything from clothing to groceries. It reminded me of Walmart except the checkout lines made the ones at Walmart look like a short cut.

The grocery store we went to was interesting, to say the least. There was the standard fare we had seen at smaller markets in the area…dried duck neck and duck feet, steak and peanut butter flavored cheetos…but the meat market was certainly a reminder that we weren't in Kansas anymore. They had live frogs, live turtles (and no, they weren't for pets), fresh squid on ice and live carp in a pool (catch your own!). For lunch we and the two other families adopting through our agency decided to go to Pizza Hut. As you might guess, it certainly was not the United States version of Pizza Hut. The restaurant was quite fancy. The workers dressed very nicely and if we didn't know any better, looking at the decor we'd think we were in a bistro in downtown Chicago. The pizza wasn't the best, but they did have quite an extensive menu, including a seafood pizza with salmon and squid. We stuck with pepperoni.

In addition to the interesting sights on our trek, I was amazed at the number of people that would come up to our group to see our "babies." Many gave us a thumbs up, and many just came to pull our daughters' pant legs down to cover the skin on their legs that had become exposed. In China, even with the weather in the 60s, they bundle their children up in at least three layers of clothing until the only skin that's showing is their face. All of the children look like the little brother in the movie *A Christmas Story*. If you haven't seen it, all the babies look like miniature sumo wrestlers wearing puffy coats.

Our last day in Wuhan we had dinner at the hotel restaurant. Squid was on the menu like it was in every other restaurant we visited. So was marinated beef shark, bull's stomach in spicy sauce, roasted pigeon, baked crab in sharkskin sauce, and fried freshwater fish's head with green onion and ginger in hot pot—one of the chef's recommendations! We were chickens and ate whatever sounded most like home.

On that last day I reflected on the elderly women we encountered the day before who cried because we were adopting abandoned children. It made us kind of uncomfortable, because we really weren't there to rescue Ava. We were there adopting Ava because we felt God called us to expand our family, and the child He had chosen for us happened to have been abandoned in China. It may sound like semantics, but there really is a world of difference between the two.

We also received some of the paperwork that was processed by the Civil Affairs Bureau in Wuhan. The last line in Ava's birth certificate read "Her birth parents and the birth place are unknown." I was really saddened when I read that. Sad for Ava and sad for the millions of other kids in the world with the same unknown history. But it also made me grateful to God for giving Ava to us, and for giving us to Ava.

The Day the World Changed

*I have been driven many times upon my knees by the
overwhelming conviction that I had nowhere else to go.*
—Abraham Lincoln

Ava's early childhood was relatively mundane. She was just a normal kid doing normal kid stuff and filling our lives with joy. She was a very spirited child who was terribly timid around strangers and wonderfully quiet at school, but never stopped talking at home. She enjoyed making up dances, songs, and knock-knock jokes. She adored her brother and sister as well as her pets. At her siblings' ball games, she was quite happy keeping herself busy playing in the dirt while wearing a pretty dress. We discovered she had a natural knack for music and she quickly developed into a talented piano player.

As a young child, Ava was rarely sick. She never even had a cold until she was four years old. In addition to being in good health she was bubbly and energetic. For example, once while we were grocery shopping she had been hopping, skipping, smiling, dancing, and singing her way through the entire store in her usual high-energy way. An elderly gentleman approached us as we headed to the checkout line to tell us it gave him so much joy to see her so full of joy that he just wanted to say thank you.

Occasionally when Ava was young I found the motivation to keep a journal and, looking back, I realized she often taught me many spiritual lessons. For example, on July 19, 2010 I wrote:

Bring a Bucket

Today we ventured to a beach along Lake Michigan in New Buffalo, MI. It was a beautiful day, warm but cloudy, which gave me some piece of mind that my skin wouldn't bubble like a bad case of smallpox. During the summer I generally have a decent tan on my arms, neck and face, but when I take my shirt off it looks like I'm still wearing a white tee shirt covered in black dog hair. I can't say I have a farmers tan since I don't farm, so I guess I should call it a courtesy tan. As a courtesy to others I don't take my shirt off. I was a bit concerned when we got to the beach because the minute we dropped our stuff in the sand everybody got out of the water. I assumed they were afraid I was going to take my shirt off but then we heard the current had gotten too strong and they weren't letting people swim any more. So our time at the beach was spent, literally, on the beach. We were able to play along the shore so I sat there with Ava as we dug holes and built castles in the sand. She then grabbed her bucket and would squat down in the wet sand, lay her bucket down so that the opening was facing the water, and wait for a wave to rush in and fill her bucket. Sometimes it would take a while for the water to reach her, but there she remained, patiently resting her bucket on the sand, confident it would be filled. I'm continually amazed at the theology one can learn from a three year old. What she was doing was exactly what we should do…be patient and know that God is always there ready to pour out his grace and mercy for us. We just have to remember to bring a bucket! My little girl didn't end her lesson there though. Once her bucket had been graced with water she would pick it up, carry it over to where I was sitting, and proceed to wash my feet with the water she had received.

She brought to life the Bible passage John 13:14-15 where Jesus instructs the apostles to be servants to others, "(Jesus said) If I, therefore, the master and teacher, have washed your feet, you ought to wash one another's feet. I have given you a model to follow, so that as I have done for you, you should also do."

Life sauntered along peacefully for several years. We were happy, we were healthy, and the future seemed to be unveiling itself as we expected it would. And then, suddenly, it didn't.

Towards the end of July, 2016, we moved Brady into an apartment in Iowa City, Iowa, as he prepared to start his new life as a student at the University of Iowa. We were surprised he chose the same school as his older sister. They are nothing alike and they were interested in two completely different fields of study. Plus, what parents get so lucky to have both kids at the same university? We quickly learned it was not luck, but Divine Providence. A week later, the little sister Macy and Brady cherished was rushed to the University of Iowa Hospitals & Clinics emergency room to begin fighting for her life.

Ava started that summer with what we thought was a case of seasonal allergies. Her nose was constantly running and stuffed up. When it didn't clear up on its own, we went to the doctor and he said it was probably a sinus infection, so he prescribed some antibiotics. When that didn't work she was prescribed some

30

allergy medication, which didn't work either. Another trip to the doctor and she was given some stronger allergy medication. When the end of July rolled around and nothing had worked yet, Ava underwent a broader test for allergies. The blood test showed she was allergic to cats, and we had two of them. We finally had our answer! Or so we thought.

The last weekend in July Ava went to visit her grandmother in Indiana to spend some quality time with her before school started and to give Renae and I time to figure out what to do with our cats. Though her nose was still stuffy and runny we dropped her off on Sunday and planned on picking her up again the next weekend. That Tuesday my mother-in-law texted Renae to let her know Ava didn't look right. Her eyes seemed a little off. We assumed it was just from her eyes being watery and rubbed all the time. My mother-in-law texted again, though, a little later that day, sharing that Ava really wasn't looking right and seemed to be getting worse. She sent us a picture and Ava's left eye looked swollen. We knew something was wrong but just assumed it might be some sort of infection resulting from two months of constant allergies. We asked my mother-in-law to see if she could get Ava into a local eye doctor to check it out and we would head out that night to pick her up.

Thankfully a wonderful eye doctor made time in her already full schedule to look at Ava. After seeing her she called us and recommended taking Ava to the emergency room. We had just gotten home from work so we packed an overnight bag and drove to meet Ava and her grandma in the emergency room in Munster, Indiana. We anticipated Ava probably getting some antibiotics and being able to come home the next day.

When we arrived in the ER at about 9:00PM on Tuesday night we were shocked when we saw Ava. She was lying in a hospital bed and her left eye was protruding from its socket, completely uneven with her right eye. We couldn't believe this was the little girl we had dropped off just forty-eight hours earlier. After we talked to Ava for a little bit the nurse asked us to follow her to another room. We knew they don't take you away to a separate room to tell you everything is OK. A short while later the doctor came in, sat down, took a deep breath, and said three terrifying words, "It's not good."

He showed us the CT (Computerized Tomography) scan they had done and it revealed an enormous tumor behind Ava's eye. It had been growing in her sinus cavity undetected until then. He could not tell us what kind of tumor it was or where all it was lodged. He couldn't tell if it was in Ava's brain, within her eye or anywhere else without doing additional testing. He informed us she needed a higher level of care than they could provide so he asked if we wanted to go to St. Francis Medical Center in Peoria, Illinois, or the Children's Hospital in Iowa City, Iowa. We chose Iowa City. Renae and Ava were immediately put in an ambulance and took off on the four hour ride to the Children's Hospital. I sped on ahead in our car. I was worn out, and a little surprised I didn't fall asleep along the way, but the shock of what we just found out kept me wide awake. The only other thing I remember about my trip was helping someone jump start their car when I stopped to get gas. I was tempted to ignore them in light of my situation, but I knew I was well ahead of the ambulance so I had no good excuse not to help. I figured it might help with karma too.

We arrived in Iowa City at about 4AM that morning and knew we were saying goodbye to our normal life. Within the first several hours Ava underwent a battery of tests and met at least two dozen different specialists and caregivers. The barrage continued for days.

Our first week at the hospital was a continuous parade of bad news. The bright spot was that an MRI (Magnetic Resonance Imaging) showed Ava's tumor had not gone into her brain or affected her eyesight. The tumor had basically reached her optic nerve but had not yet caused any issues. In fact, one of the times Ava was reading letters on a card for the eye doctor, the doctor had a puzzled look on his face and asked what she was reading. She pointed to one of the small rows at the bottom of the card—one the doctor could barely see!

Doctors, of course, needed a biopsy of the tumor so Ava was taken into surgery for that and a buffet of other procedures. Thankfully they didn't have to do any cutting on her head or face to get the tissue sample they needed. They just ended up spelunking through her left nostril. That was great, except once she was out of surgery her nose wouldn't stop bleeding. They eventually halted the flow by spraying a concoction up her nose that reminded me of the expandable foam I use to fill gaps in my house. While she was under anesthesia they also inserted a needle into her hip bone to withdraw some bone marrow for testing. She had a gastronomy tube (g-tube) placed into her stomach to help with nutrition and a port implanted in her chest to receive chemotherapy. The procedures took several hours to complete, and then another hour or so waiting for the anesthesia to wear off. It was an extremely long and painful day.

After the tumor was biopsied we anxiously awaited the results. Due to the pathologist's schedule and a weekend thrown in the mix, we had to wait almost a week for the findings. They say patience is a virtue, but they also say a dog's mouth is cleaner than a human's, and my dog eats her own poop. Doctors told us it was going to be one of two types of cancer, and one was easier to treat than the other. Ava's, we found out, was the harder one to treat called rhabdomyosarcoma, an aggressive soft-tissue cancer with no clearly known cause. Then we were told there are two variations of rhabdomyosarcoma. One has better outcomes than the other. Yep, she had alveolar rhabdomyosarcoma which had the lower chance for a positive outcome. We've always told Ava she was one in a million and, statistically, we were correct. Alveolar Rhabdomyosarcoma occurs in one of every one million children.

By this time we dreaded when the doctors came in because the news just kept getting worse. And it did get worse. A lot worse. We learned the cancer was considered stage IV because it had already spread from her sinus cavity to her spine, ribs, and bone marrow. I remember thinking this has to be the worst news any parent could ever hear. Then, in a weirdly comforting way I thought no, the worst news a parent could hear would have to be their child is missing, so I couldn't really complain too much. We were just grateful Ava was not in any pain. Being a nurse, Renae knew doctors sometimes do not give patients the whole truth about their condition. We wanted the truth and she bluntly asked if treating Ava had the possibility of a positive outcome or were we just going to be putting her through hell to put off the inevitable. Our doctor was very understanding and reassured us that Ava had a chance of getting through this. Then, at our request, he gave us the grim statistic. Because Ava's cancer had metastasized to so many locations, she was considered to be in the "High Risk" group. He said the five year survival rate (the percentage of children alive five years after diagnosis) for a child with rhabdomyosarcoma in the High Risk group is around thirty percent. On the one hand, the news was terrible. The odds were definitely not in our favor. On the other hand, I was expecting him to give us a survival rate in the single digits, so again I was grateful. She was going to be in for a very tough battle, but we were thankful she had a chance.

Illness & Treatment

When you come to the end of all the light you know, and it's time to step into the darkness of the unknown, faith is knowing that one of two things shall happen: Either you will be given something solid to stand on or you will be taught to fly.
—Edward Teller

Ava is a deeply introspective child and often hits me, usually when she's supposed to be going to bed, with profound theological questions. She's always had a curiosity about God and faith and, particularly, about Heaven. "What's it like? Why do we have to live here first before going there? Why would someone not get to go there? Will there be school there since I haven't finished it down here? Will it have rainbows?" are just a few of her inquiries. One of my first thoughts after her diagnosis was that now she might get her answers.

During a couple of low points she confessed she was tired of being sick, tired of having cancer and just wanted to go to heaven. To say that was hard to hear is putting it mildly. The most difficult question Ava posed came a week after her treatment started. With tears streaming she asked, "Daddy, not to be rude, but why does God want me to suffer? I've never been a bully to anyone!" I think I muddled through a response about God allowing suffering to bring about a greater good, though I found it hard to understand myself when looking at my suffering daughter's tears. I know God only gives gifts, but I was having a hard time unwrapping this one.

Ava's original treatment plan was scheduled to last fifty-four weeks. Most of those weeks involved us driving sixty miles from our home to the hospital in Iowa City for chemo treatments which lasted anywhere from a few minutes to an entire week. On her first day of treatment she heard the doctors talk to Renae about chemotherapy's possible side-effects. Later that day she tearfully confessed that hearing them talk scared her and she didn't want to die. All I could think was I couldn't believe I was having this conversation with my nine year old daughter. I tried to reassure her by saying some of the best doctors in the world are working together to make her better, and I prayed they would.

The treatment plan seemed to go well at first. Ava would finish an infusion and be ready to head back to school the next day. Except for her bald head you couldn't tell she was in a fight for her life. This was pretty much the case until she completed her radiation treatments in February of 2017. In addition to chemo she had radiation treatments on several sites in her body every day for five and a half weeks. This intense regimen took a terrible toll on her immune system. She was no longer able to bounce right back after chemo treatments. Her blood counts (white blood cells, platelets, hemoglobin, etc.) would become dangerously low and lead to other serious problems. With counts so low, we would postpone upcoming rounds of chemo until her blood counts recovered, which could take several weeks. We were told administering chemo with low blood counts could tax her bone marrow past the point of no return. Her counts would no longer be able to recover so then she would need a bone marrow transplant. Obviously something we didn't want her to have to go through. So, we had to agonizingly wait for her tiny little body to recover on its own. While we would wait, her low counts would frequently cause her to develop a fever (called a neutropenic fever) which meant she had to be admitted into the hospital and stay there for several days. Often she received blood transfusions to keep her energy up while we were waiting for her own blood to bounce back. The first time she received a transfusion she was a bit concerned and asked if she was getting a boy's blood. The doctor assured her they test for cooties so she had nothing to worry about. She smiled at the good news.

Prior to her series of radiation treatments, Ava would often feel tired and sometimes nauseated after chemotherapy, but those were generally the only side effects she experienced. It didn't help that one of the chemo drugs she received in the hospital is very toxic to the kidneys so they pumped her full of fluids and made her go to the bathroom every two hours during her stay. It's hard not to be tired when a nurse wakes you every two hours throughout the night to pee.

The postponement of her scheduled chemos caused no little anxiety for Renae and I. Though the doctors said delays were common, all we could think about was the cancer cells taking advantage of the cease fire—regrouping, and coming back even stronger. The doctors eventually prescribed medicine to help Ava's blood counts recover faster and thankfully the cancer never spread beyond its original locations. The medicine was a stress-inducing shot we had to give after most of her remaining rounds of chemo. Stress inducing because we had to give it to her at home twenty-four hours after the completion of an infusion. "We" meant Renae, of course. Renae had given many shots in her nursing career without thinking twice about it. However, when it is your child, and the shot costs around $14,000, and you have to shoot the medicine from a pre-filled syringe into a sterile vial then draw out the exact amount needed with a different syringe, then inject it into a pinch of fat that your child does not have, it becomes next-level.

We were so proud how Ava faced this and all of the other necessary brutality she had to endure. When she was younger it took a roll of duct tape, three nurses, and a WWF wrestler to hold her down for a shot. Even when she gave blood for her allergy test a few weeks before her diagnosis she was sweating profusely and needed us to sit next to her to comfort her. In her treatment she became a warrior princess. She had so many shots, blood draws and IVs but since she knew she needed them she put on a brave face and bit the bullet. This was no easy task, especially later on in her treatment. Her blood draws started resembling a type of medieval torture as it became harder for nurses and phlebotomists to connect with her veins. They would start in one arm, unsuccessfully dig around for a while with the needle inside her and conclude they need to try the other arm instead. Sometimes digging around in the other arm didn't work either so they would stab the end of her finger and milk the blood from it like a cow. It was a terrible thing to watch, but at the same time I was so proud of how tough my little girl was. With teeth clenched and tears running down her face she would sit still, taking it like a war hero being tortured for vital information.

The irony was not lost on Ava that it was not cancer that made her feel terrible but her treatments. Once Ava started struggling with her blood counts, chemotherapy's side effects began rearing their ugly head. She lost her sense of taste, which is not a great situation for someone already eating like Gandhi. On several occasions she developed mucositis. Mucositis is a horribly painful condition where your mouth and GI tract fill with ulcers and you salivate profusely, making it hard to eat or talk. It was as delightful for her as it sounds. Thankfully Renae had the foresight before treatments began to request that Ava have a G-tube surgically inserted into her stomach. Ava was already rail-thin and a picky eater before diagnosis and we knew things were only going to get worse. And they did.

In April, 2017 an echocardiogram showed her port, for some unexplained reason, had moved. A port is a nickel-sized disc implanted into the chest just under the skin with a catheter that connects it to a large vein. An IV is stuck into the disk to administer chemo drugs, among other things. Ava's port movement caused the catheter to actually touch one of her heart valves. This could have caused serious complications so she had to have surgery to repair it.

In May Ava developed swelling in her left cheek near her eye… close to the same spot of her original tumor. She looked like she had been in a fight and lost. An MRI was done and the results came back inconclusive. We were told the swelling was either caused by her tumor starting to grow again or due to faulty sinus drainage resulting from the radiation she had received in her cheek. Doctors treated both scenarios and an MRI a couple of weeks later thankfully showed the swelling was just caused by an abscess in her cheek.

July was a pretty rough month. A couple of ER visits due to fevers, a urinary tract infection, mucositis, surgery to drain the abscess and implant a stent into her tear duct to improve drainage, X-rays, a PET (Positron Emission Tomography) scan, blood and platelet transfusions, chemo. After spending twenty-four days in the hospital that month, she was just plain sick of being there. The months were surely testing all of us.

In early November, 2017 we traveled to Iowa City for one of Ava's last rounds of chemo. It was not an infusion that required her blood counts to be at a certain level, but she'd had an infusion the prior week her counts were pretty dismal. Because of her poor blood counts we stayed a couple hours longer so she could receive a blood transfusion, which was not uncommon. However, by the time the transfusion finished, Ava developed a fever which meant our few hours appointment had just turned into at least a few days. That week in the hospital she developed typhlitis, a potentially fatal bacterial infection caused by her chemotherapy drugs damaging her intestinal lining. Her fever, heart rate and stomach contents went up and her blood pressure went down so they admitted her into the pediatric intensive care unit (PICU). We couldn't believe we were so close to being done with treatment and here she was in a brand new battle for survival. Thankfully they were able to stabilize her in the PICU and she only had to stay there one night. She was finally released from the hospital the day before Thanksgiving. We had so much to be thankful for that day.

On December 11th, 2017, more than 18 months after diagnosis, Ava received her last chemotherapy infusion! It was a great and joyful day, one we thought would never arrive. The joy did not last long though. Apparently Ava liked typhlitis so much, three days after her last chemo she decided to get it again. She ended up in the PICU once more, this time for two nights. She was in terrible pain for a long time but thankfully was able to come home from the hospital just before Christmas.

During her last month of treatment Ava spent 25 nights in the hospital. Over her entire treatment span she amassed over 130 nights in the hospital, 150 blood draws, 200 doses of radiation, 60 clinic visits, 35 rounds of chemo, 34 shots, 8 blood transfusions, and well over a thousand doses of medicine. It's amazing her little body tolerated all that was done to her, yet she could still light up a room when she smiled.

Because the shots to stimulate Ava's blood counts could produce a false positive on her end-of-treatment MRI, we had to wait a month before we could find out if her treatments actually worked. Though we were incredibly anxious to find out the results, we were OK with having to wait until after Christmas. If it was going to be bad news at least we could enjoy the holiday.

When the day finally arrived for the scans to see how her cancer responded, I was a stomach knot wrapped inside a bundle of nerves sprinkled with a ray of hope. I tried to stay positive. We wanted Ava to be over this so badly. She had been through so much already I didn't think I'd be able to watch her go through more or that her little body could handle any more. After her scans she was taken to a recovery room while we waited for the anesthesia to wear off. She'd been anesthetized several times before without incident but this time was different. As she floated into consciousness her body started shaking, her voice was hoarse, her breathing was abnormal and she couldn't open her eyes. These, plus the fact that she was still loopy from the anesthesia, caused her to cry and scream uncontrollably. There was nothing we could do to console her. We were in the basement of the hospital and were pretty sure the kids on the 11th floor could hear her. As we unsuccessfully tried to calm her the oncologist stopped by to give us the results. With a big smile he shared that no cancer had been detected! The cancer was in remission! The prayers we and so many other people had prayed had been answered! Praise God!

We danced for joy, threw confetti, and shouted cries of thanksgiving at the top of our lungs. Ok, not really. That was how we imagined that day would be, but with Ava screaming teamed with our immediate concern for her, the moment we had waited a year-and-a-half for became an anticlimactic but extremely heartfelt and joyful thank you to him (and Him). By the time we got home Ava had finally come back to her normal state and we were able to smother her with hugs and kisses for the first time in a long time as a child without cancer.

Photos

*Life with God is not immunity from difficulties,
but peace in difficulties.*—C.S. Lewis

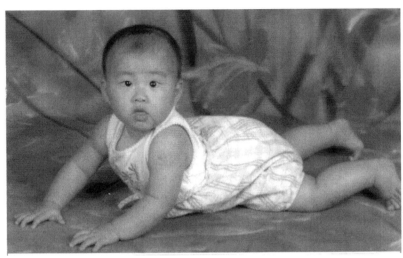

The first picture we received of Ava as part of her referral packet from China.

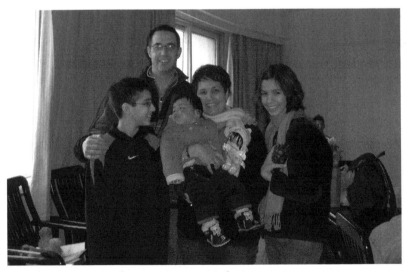

Gotcha Day! Our first moments with Ava.

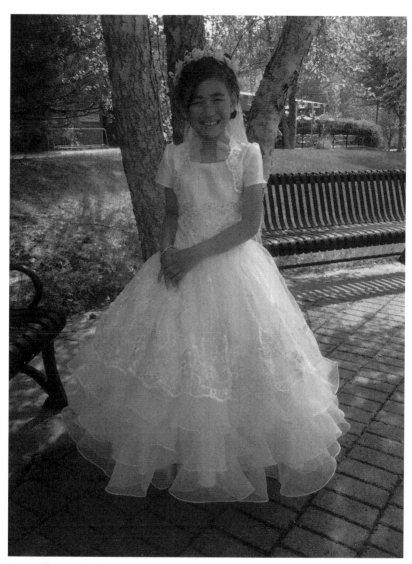

Proudly modeling her First Communion Dress.

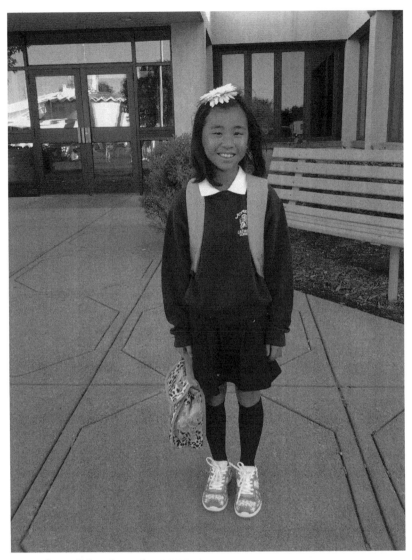

First day of third grade, 2015.

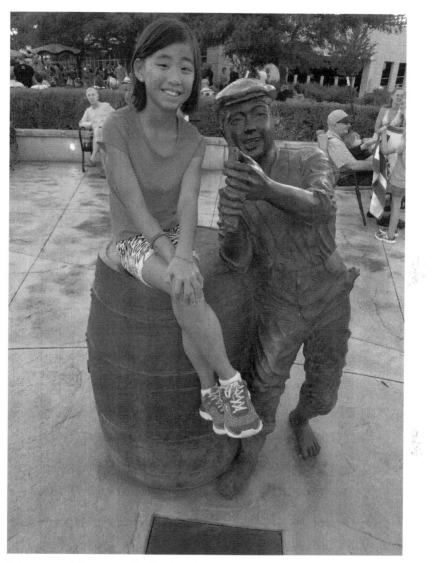

July 2016. Three weeks before being rushed to the hospital.

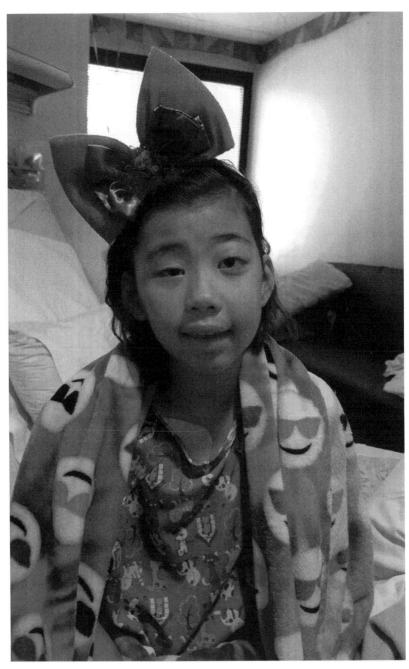

First week in the children's hospital. Newly diagnosed but still stylin'.

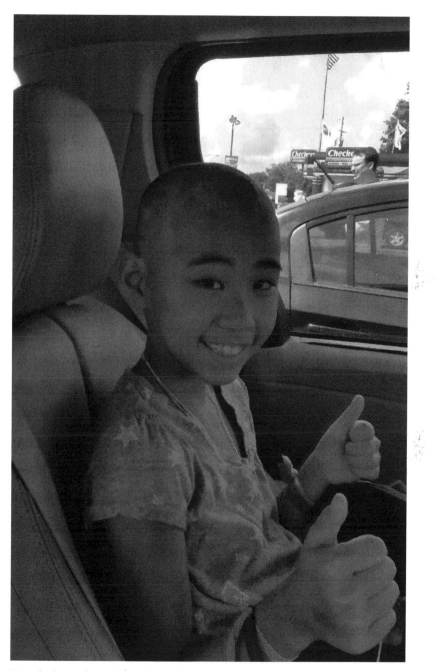

Head shaved and ready to fight the good fight!

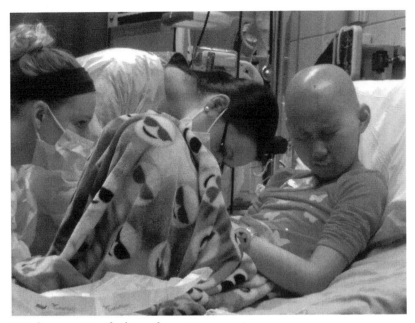

Finding a vein, feeling the pain….again.

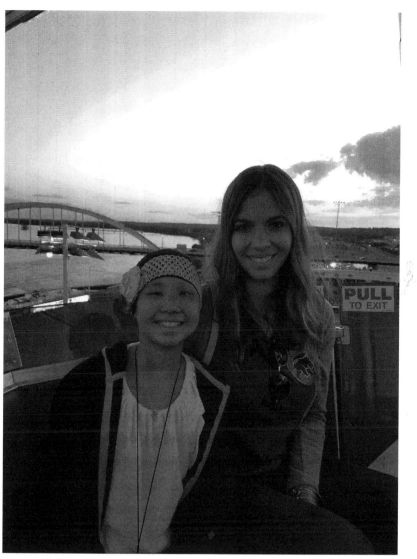

Ava and Macy enjoying a ferris wheel ride above the Mississippi River.

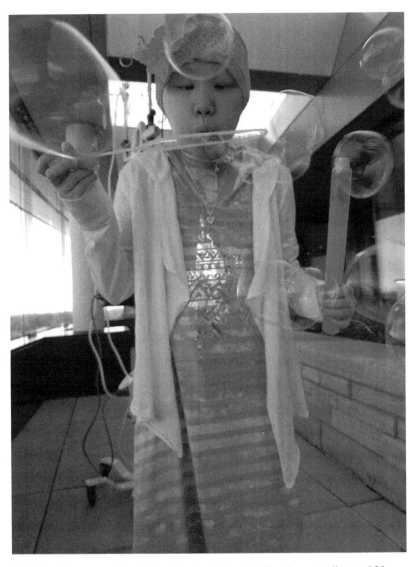

Making her own fun blowing bubbles in the hospital's twelfth floor open-air garden.

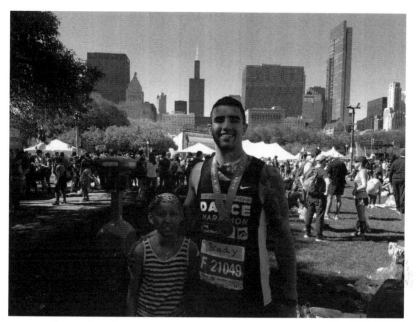

Ava and Brady after he ran the Chicago Marathon for her and her fellow patients.

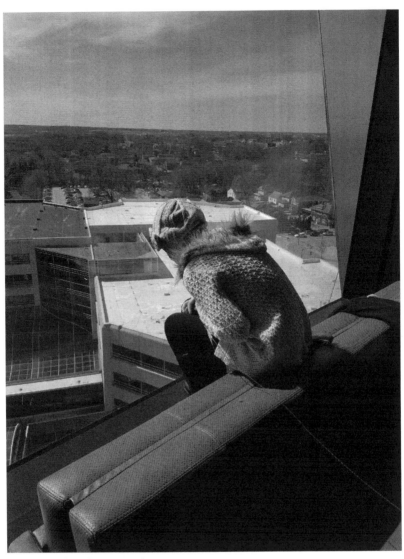

Longing for the outside

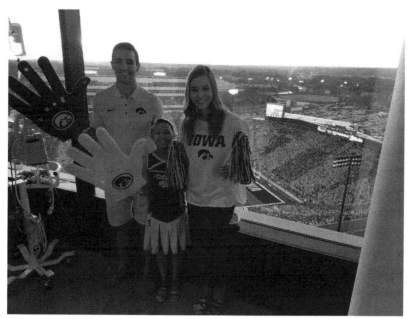

Armed and ready to wave back.

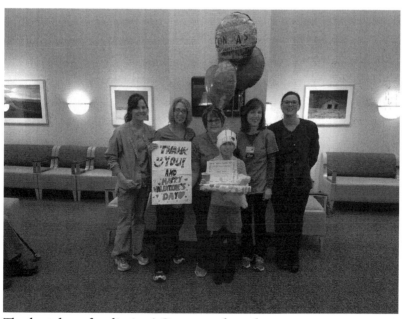

The last day of radiation! Or so we thought.

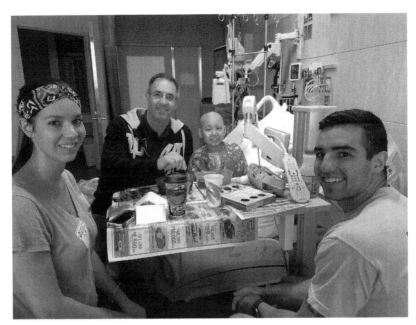

Decorating eggs for Easter.

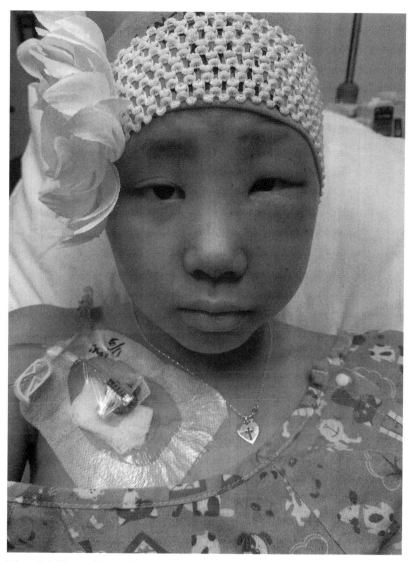

Thankfully only an abscess under her eye and not her cancer spreading.

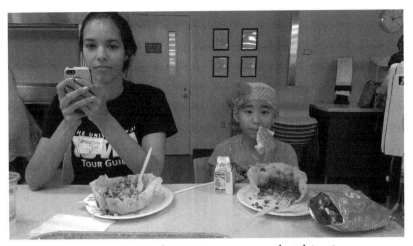

Thanks to appetite stimulants, Ava out-eats her big sister.

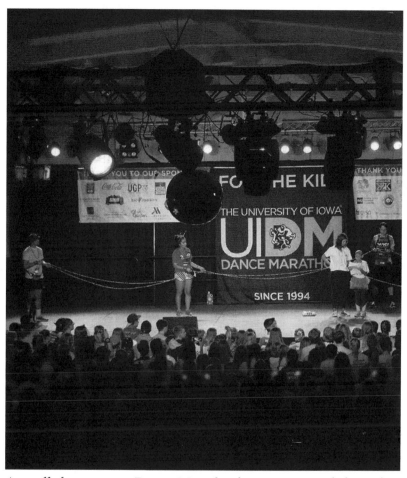

Ava tells her story at Dance Marathon's Big Event and shows her string of bravery beads.

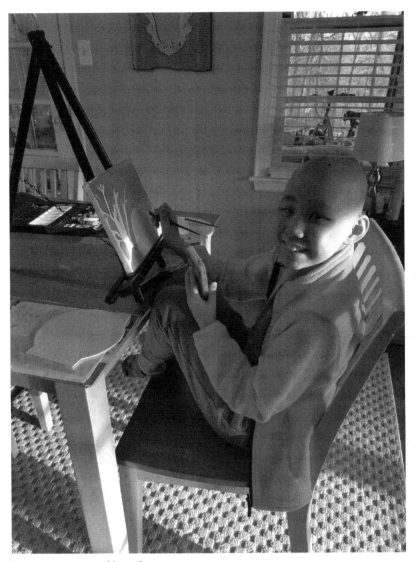

Enjoying one of her favorite pastimes.

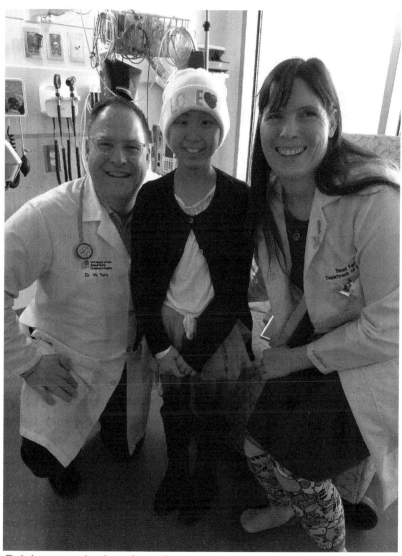

Celebrating the last day of chemo with her two amazing doctors
Dr. Terry and Dr. Truscott.

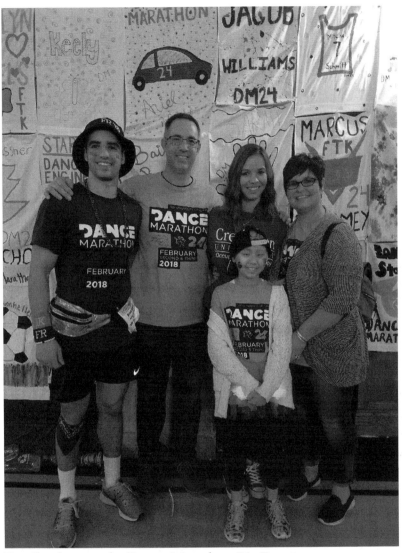

Family photo at the Dance Marathon Big Event.

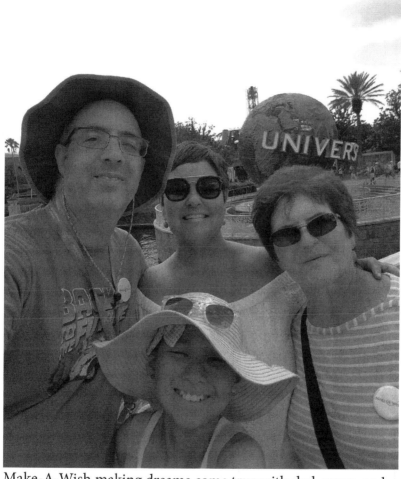

Make-A-Wish making dreams come true with dad, mom, and grandma at Universal Studios.

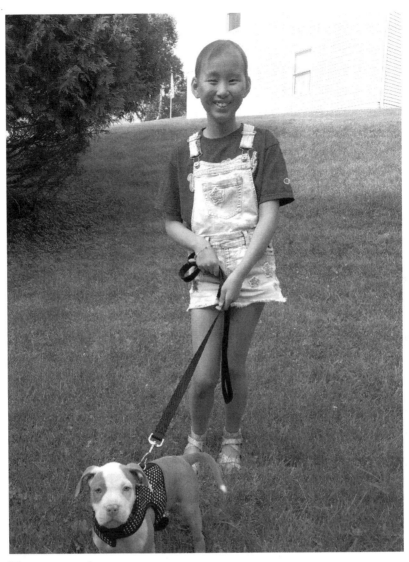

The promised puppy.

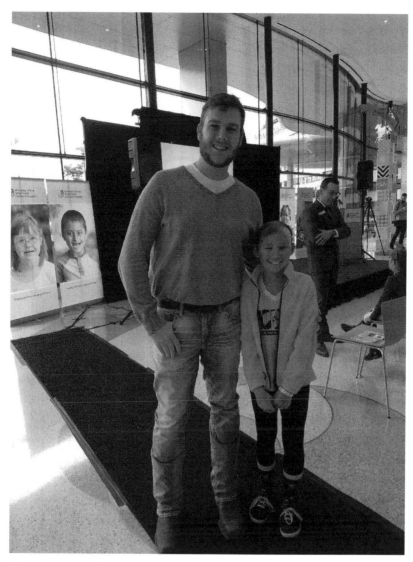

Meeting Mr. Carson King the day he donated $3 million to the Stead Family Children's Hospital.

Where Was God?

God is love
—1 John 4:8

As Jesus hung on the cross in agony, the Bible says he uttered seven final statements. A last will and testament of sorts. At one point he cried out the words of verse 2 from Psalm 22, "My God, my God, why have you abandoned me?" In the midst of Ava's illness Jesus' cry became very real to me. Where was he in all of this? I always assumed Jesus was quoting this verse to describe his physical pain and loneliness on the cross. But as I reflected on these words during Ava's battle, I began to believe He also asked this because it is the one question every human being asks at one time or another, in one form or another—

"God, why did this happen?"

"How could you do that?"

"What am I going to do now?"

"I don't deserve this!"

These are all variations of that cry and by reciting it, Jesus let each of us know that no matter what we face, He knows how we feel and is helping us through it. Though it starts as a cry of despair, Psalm 22 concludes as an answered prayer: "For he has not spurned or disdained the misery of this poor wretch, Did not turn away from me, but heard me when I cried out."-Psalm 22:25

I've never really found it very hard to pray. Not to say I've always done it or I'm very good at it, but in most of my adult life I've generally found it easy to converse with God. Of course, a lot of times it's been in the format of an employee performance review. "God, you did pretty well in these areas last week but here's what I'd like you to do for me now." After Ava's diagnosis however, I was surprised I didn't know what to say to God. I wasn't mad, even though I thought I should be. I think I was just so stunned I didn't know what to say. Several years ago after Mother Teresa of Calcutta passed away, some of her writings were uncovered and revealed that she often felt as if God were absent from her life. I thought maybe this is how she felt during those dark times. As my prayer life slowly began to return, I started asking, "God, where are you?" Though Mother Teresa eventually understood her darkness as a way for her to be united to Christ's abandonment on the Cross, I believe God just wanted to make sure I was paying attention when he showed my family all of the ways he was making himself present during Ava's illness.

Though I didn't recognize them initially, eventually my eyes were opened to the many gifts of God's presence on our journey. The first was the fact that, though Ava had been one of hundreds of thousands of orphans in China, she now happened to be a beloved child in a family that lived an hour away from one of the world's premier pediatric cancer centers. There is no way she would have been given the treatment she needed had she still lived in China. The second occurred shortly after Ava was admitted on our first day in the hospital. A parade of white coats entered the room and introduced themselves as Ava's care team. There must have been a dozen doctors, nurses and other caregivers letting us know they were there to help us through this. Their presence was both frightening and reassuring. Frightening because so many people were needed to take care of Ava, but reassuring because she had so many good people caring for her and dedicated to making our daughter well. I strongly believe each one of them was, and is, a gift from God. From that point on we were surrounded by so much love we could barely comprehend it. Love came at us from every direction and in many unexpected ways.

CARE TEAM/HOSPITAL STAFF

During our first meeting with Ava's care team, one of our nurse practitioners urged us to let people help while our world was being turned upside down. My initial thought was "Yeah OK whatever. I see your lips moving but all I hear is blah, blah, blah." Renae and I take pride in doing things on our own and don't like to burden people with our problems. They've got enough of their own to worry about. We were going to be fine and weren't going to bother anyone else. Then came the Slurpee.

One warm day after school while Ava was in-between chemotherapy cycles she wanted to stop at a local gas station to get a Slurpee. When we got to the counter the clerk noticed Ava with no hair and generously said to go ahead, the Slurpee was on her. I thanked her but insisted I pay for it. I handed her the money and as we walked back to the car this overwhelming feeling of guilt poured over me. I thought of how good it makes me feel when I do something nice for someone, and I realized I had just deprived the clerk of the joy of doing something nice for Ava. I also deprived Ava the joy of experiencing someone doing something nice for her. I was a big fat roadblock preventing a simple expression of love. I vowed from that point on to get out of the way and let people help us whenever they felt moved to do so. I'm glad I did because we absolutely needed it and help was on the way.

One of my favorite movie scenes of all time, right up there with the bean scene from *Blazing Saddles* and anything from National Lampoon's *Christmas Vacation* or *Monty Python and the Holy Grail*, is from the movie *Miracle on the Hudson*. In the scene, Pilot Chesley "Sully" Sullenberger is being accused by the National Transportation Safety Board (NTSB) of not responding appropriately after his aircraft lost both engines at an altitude lower than any jet in history due to a bird strike. The NTSB's computer simulations showed he had time to get to a runway instead of landing in the Hudson River. After hearing the NTSB's case, Sully leans forward and sternly but calmly asks, "Can we get serious now?" He asked how many times the pilot in the simulation practiced that maneuver before it was successful. Seventeen times! Sully scolded the NTSB because their simulation did not account for the human factor, the time it took to analyze the unprecedented situation. This was an event that no pilot had ever trained for or encountered. Within seconds the seasoned pilot had to analyze the jet's condition, altitude, speed, locations of nearby airports, the presence of people and structures on the ground between them and the airports, and the potential for loss of life in all possible scenarios. Considering these data points, he decided the best chance for survival was to land the powerless jet into the frigid Hudson River. Every one of the 155 people on board survived that day and Sully was rightly declared a hero. Watching that scene makes me think of Ava's oncologists. Each day for them was an unprecedented situation with a life hanging in the balance. The side effects of chemo drugs, current prescriptions, medical history, radiation schedule, blood test results, fevers, infections, weight, temperature, appetite, kidney function, heart function, and her body's reactions to all of the above had to be constantly monitored because at a given moment any one or combination of those things could go south, as they often did. The oncologists had to quickly respond each time to avert potentially tragic consequences. I am so grateful to Dr. William Terry, Dr. Jamie Truscott, and the rest of Ava's care team for answering their call to the ministry of pediatric oncology. We will never be able repay them for giving us our daughter back.

Nurses are a special breed, and pediatric oncology nurses are arguably the most special of all. We were so blessed by all of the nurses that took care of Ava. Whether in the outpatient clinic or in a hospital room, they made us feel like Ava was their only patient and they cared for her as if she were one of their own family members. They were always smiling and cheerful and willing to do anything we needed to make our visits better. It almost made us wonder what kind of "medicine" they were keeping in the nurse's lounge. Even though most of the time they came into the room amidst the cloud of administering chemo or making Ava use the bathroom or giving her other medicine, they always brought a cloud-dispersing sunshine with them.

An example that really exemplifies this occurred one Saturday afternoon in 2018 during the Iowa Hawkeye football season. There was a home game and, as is well-known now, kids and their families were invited to the top floor of the hospital to watch. Unfortunately, because Ava had to be kept isolated from others at the time we were unable to join the festivities. To make things worse, the only thing we could see from her room was a corner of the scoreboard in Kinnick Stadium. We were so close yet so far away. About an hour before the game started our nurse came into our room and said, "If you don't mind, I went ahead and moved

Ava's room to an empty one closer to the stadium so you can watch the game."

We smiled. "If we don't mind!?" In two minutes we were packed up and ready to relocate. The gesture made an unfortunate situation quite enjoyable. The view was phenomenal and we felt like we were watching the game in a luxury box suite...minus the alcohol of course. The nurses' daily unselfish and loving service to our family made a tremendous difference in our lives, brought joy to our sorrow, and we will never forget them.

Along with the standard doctor and nurse types, Stead Family Children's Hospital also employs people whose job it is to help comfort the kids during their hospital visits. These saintly people are called Childlife Specialists. They have answered a call to help make a child's hospital experience less traumatic. They are there to comfort children whether they are anxious about a needle stick, terrified of an upcoming surgery, or just bored being in the hospital. We leaned on them pretty heavily at the beginning of Ava's hospital visits to help soothe her dislike of sharp metal objects being thrust into her skin. As Ava became more accustomed to being hygienically stabbed, we relied more on their other skill set...having fun with kids. They provided Ava with games and puzzles, arts and crafts, and her favorite, TV bingo. The Childlife Specialists would be on the hospital TV and play bingo with any kids in the hospital that were interested. Winners, and there were many, would get to choose a prize from the prize cart they wheeled around after the game. Ava loved winning bingo prizes and cherished her Childlife angels.

Not surprisingly, Ava wasn't normally very interested in doing things when she was getting chemo in the hospital. It appears having your body filled with horribly toxic chemicals tends to decrease your desire for frolicking and socializing. I'm sure the government has spent millions of dollars confirming this. There was one thing that Ava was always up for though, no matter how bad she felt—art. The hospital provides an art therapist and, even on her worst days, when the art therapist came by the room Ava would perk up and create something beautiful with her. We are so grateful Ava had this bright spot in her disassociated life, this one thing that always made her happy.

When I watched Ava enjoy creating art in the midst of an otherwise unenjoyable situation, I thought how tragic it is when schools cut art programs when money gets tight. I saw first hand how art can speak to a child when other things do not. Art often enters the side door when kids are not answering the front door, and I know many kids have no interest in answering the front door at all.

PRAYER

One of the first emails I sent after Ava's diagnosis was to our parish's (St. Pius X Catholic Church in Rock Island, IL) prayer chain. I knew Ava was in need of an army of prayer warriors to fight alongside her. Many people in the chain forwarded Ava's needs to their friends on other prayer chains as well. Prayer chain people usually can't keep prayer needs to themselves or belong to just one. They understand prayer's economy of scale. Each prayer they and so many others offered for us was a hand that helped us bear the weight of the very heavy cross we were carrying.

During our initial two-week stay in the hospital we were able to get out of the room every once in a while so we would walk around to explore—as much as you can explore with a child wearing a mask and connected to an IV pole. I'll never forget entering one of the elevators in the main hospital. It was a little crowded and Ava ended up standing next to a petite older woman. As the door closed I noticed the woman raise her hand up over Ava, close her eyes and lift her head toward heaven in silent prayer. I was in awe. She had no idea who my daughter was or what was wrong with her but she loved her anyway. I wish I would have thanked her for the prayer. Instead, I just stood there, amazed and grateful. Her small gesture was a priceless gift. It was the first time I sensed we might get through this.

As time went on so many people let us know they were praying and offering Masses for us. One of Ava's teachers sent out a prayer request to over two hundred of her friends and family to pray for Ava. She had people from all over the world...USA, Italy, France, and Africa...praying, including communities of nuns in Illinois and France. A few months later her teacher she took a trip to Italy and prayed for us at each church and holy place she visited, including the tomb of St. Francis of Assisi. She even had the privilege of attending an audience with Pope Francis and came to the hospital when she returned to give Ava a medal and bracelet blessed by him.

We were blessed to have Fr. Ted Hochstatter praying for us, a friend and former associate pastor at our parish. He has spent years working with Mother Teresa's Sisters of Charity in Africa's largest slum. Daily he was surrounded by immense suffering but he made time to help alleviate ours and sent us emails on more than one occasion to let us know he and the people of his parish were praying for us.

Friends of ours visited The National Shrine of Our Lady of Good Help near Green Bay, Wisconsin, dedicated to the only Catholic Church approved Marian apparition site in the United

States. They brought home a small container of holy water from there and gave it to us. I was already placing my hand on Ava's head to give her a blessing before she went to bed and making the sign of the cross on her forehead. After receiving the holy water I added the water to my thumb when making the sign of the cross each night. I felt all of heaven was with me as I blessed her. Ava sometimes would even return the favor and bless me with it.

For many years I have visited our parish's perpetual adoration chapel one hour each week to pray. A perpetual adoration chapel is a beautifully peaceful place where, as Catholics, we believe Jesus Christ is actually present in the Eucharist, body, blood, soul, and divinity, twenty-four hours a day, seven days a week, three hundred sixty-five days a year. I, and many others, experience it as a place where we can pour out our heart and have it filled, all at the same time. I can honestly say my hour there is the best hour of my week.

Though there were many weeks I was unable to go due to Ava's hospitalizations, I had wonderful friends that joyfully went in my stead to pray. Surprisingly, when we weren't at the hospital and I was able to get to the chapel, I sometimes found it quite difficult to pray. I found it hard to articulate what I wanted to say to Jesus. After a while of struggling with words, I asked his mother, Mary, to help me pray. In time, an image emerged in my mind of what I had such a hard time trying to say. I pictured my frail, bald, sick little girl cradled in the arms of the Blessed Mother, who was standing next to Jesus. She was holding Ava against his Sacred Heart while he placed his healing hand on her head. This image gave me great comfort and reminded me of the hospital priest who at the beginning reassured us Jesus is the lead physician in charge of Ava's care. Jesus was Ava's physician while Mary was a nurse to my soul.

Soon after our initial hospital stay we received a card in the mail from the Sisters of St. Francis of the Martyr St. George, an order of nuns that teach at Ava's school and have a convent at our parish. They assured us of their prayers, informing us they were offering a rosary novena and asking the intercession of Fr. Edward Flanagan for Ava's healing. A rosary is a prayer of prayers really. One basically prays an Our Father prayer followed by ten Hail Mary prayers (called a "decade"), and this is done five times. Each decade is spent reflecting on a different aspect of Jesus' life while you pray. There are a few other prayers sprinkled in as well but the Our Fathers and Hail Marys are the meat of it. A novena just means they would be praying these particular prayers specifically for Ava for nine consecutive days. It meant so much to us that the sisters were thinking of Ava and offering prayers for her, and we were amazed they asked Fr. Flanagan to intercede on her behalf as well. They happened to choose him because some of the sisters had recently visited Boys Town, Nebraska, where he had dedicated his life helping orphans. Coincidentally the sisters were asking him to pray with them for a little girl that used to be an orphan herself. We knew Ava was in good hands.

FAMILY AND FRIENDS

One of our first gifts of hope was from a wonderful friend whose two oldest children are twins, a boy and a girl, that went to high school with our daughter Macy. Macy and her daughter are close friends. The twin son happened to have been diagnosed with the same kind of cancer as Ava a couple of years earlier and was in remission. Having already been through the ordeal of a child with cancer, she wanted to ease our anxiety and put together a folder with several positive stories of rhabdomyosarcoma survivors including one of a local high school state championship wrestler, diagnosed in 2014, who recently completed treatments and was in remission. I can't begin to tell you what a difference this made. She gave us a great sense of hope, especially at a time when we weren't feeling very hopeful.

The funny thing about a disease completely redirecting the course of your life is that life in the rest of the world keeps marching along as if nothing happened. There is still work to attend to, bills to pay, a house to maintain, and, as in our case, our other kids we didn't want to leave behind. My mother-in-law often made the four hour trip to Iowa City from Indiana to stay with Ava so Renae and I could go to work and take care of some of those other things that needed our attention. We really appreciated her enabling us to stay relatively connected to our jobs and other responsibilities as well as give Ava an occasional break from us. I'm sure Ava appreciated that and we are eternally indebted to her for all she did for us.

During Ava's first couple of weeks in the hospital I headed home one afternoon to take care of some things around the house, including mowing the lawn. The whole drive home I was dreading mowing. Our yard isn't that big but it's very hilly, rather treacherous in places—simply put, it's not easy to mow. Throw in the heat of early August and the fact that life had just smacked me in the gut like Babe Ruth swinging a Louisville Slugger, and I wasn't quite feeling up to it. It's probably the first time I ever drove the actual speed limit on I-80. Once I finally reached home I turned into the driveway and...wow, my yard was completely mowed! I was shocked and, of course, thrilled. The person who mowed it was still there but it wasn't anyone I knew. I could tell he worked for a lawn service so I asked who put him up to it. He said he wasn't supposed to tell me. After much cajoling on my part he finally gave up that it was our next-door neighbor. This was such a wonderful gift, just one less thing to worry about while we were worrying about Ava. Many other friends brought meals over since grocery shopping and cooking had moved pretty far down our priority list. Many other family and friends were there to help us in whatever way we needed. Lots of prayers, gifts, gas cards, food gift cards, emails, and visits helped bring light to our darkness. We were incredibly blessed to be surrounded by so much kindness. They were all a living parable to our family: "Amen, I say to you, whatever you did for one of these least brothers of mine, you did for me." Matthew 25:40

SCHOOL AND WORK

Before we could even wrap our heads around what was happening with Ava we were smothered with the generosity of our work and school communities. At Ava's school (Jordan Catholic School) and Renae's work (UnityPoint Health), orders were being taken for a "Team Ava" shirt and bracelet fundraiser. My co-workers at the Rock Island-Milan School District had collected donations for our family, making sure there was at least enough money for Ava to get an iPad so she wouldn't be so bored at the hospital.

Our employers were incredibly sympathetic and understanding of our "new normal," as Ava's oncologist called it. I can't imagine a parent going through what we went through and not getting the level of support we received from our workplaces. I imagine that extra weight of worry could crush a person. We were so glad we didn't have to find out.

There is no way to put into words what it meant to be able to focus on Ava without the fear of being punished or losing our jobs. We worked as much as possible, both to try and keep up with our work loads and to give our minds something else to focus on every once in a while. Fortunately I was able to do a lot of my work online in the hospital. With as many nights Ava stayed in the hospital during her treatment, this was a tremendous help.

Generosity seemed everywhere. So many of our coworkers went above and beyond to help us in our need. It seemed they were always sending us gift cards and notes of encouragement. One of mine, in particular, committed to paying forward the joy she and her husband had received from the cards and gifts they had gotten when he underwent cancer treatment several years ago. She remembered how nice it was whenever someone sent a card or gift, so every month she sent Ava a card and gift to lift her spirits. They always seemed to come at just the right time.

Just as our employers gave us unparalleled support at work, the teachers, students, and staff at Jordan Catholic School went above and beyond making this scary experience as pleasant as possible for Ava. They let her have a Chromebook computer to use while she was confined to the hospital or home so she could keep up with her studies as much as possible (this was before COVID made online learning commonplace). One of Ava's biggest fears was falling behind and having to repeat a grade without her classmates, so this was a much appreciated gift. Her teachers were so understanding of Ava's situation and let her work at whatever pace she was able. Students and staff often made cards for Ava to cheer her up, which always did. One of her classmates even shaved his head to show his support. We all thought that was pretty cool.

In addition to supporting the Team Ava bracelet sale, Ava's classmates, their parents, and teachers organized a bake sale at school. Ava was really missing school but it gave her great joy knowing her friends were thinking of her and cared enough to organize the event. It genuinely made her feel special. We sincerely appreciated the thought and effort behind the event, as well as the donation it generated to put toward our medical expenses. In Catholic theology, actions we take that extend God's compassion to those in need fall into two categories—the Corporal (physical) Works of Mercy and the Spiritual Works of Mercy. There are few things more beautiful than children living out the Corporal Works of Mercy by giving to a family in need, as Ava's classmates did. Few things except maybe when they were living out the Spiritual Works of Mercy by praying for Ava in class.

Speaking of mercy, a few weeks after Ava's last chemo treatment I stopped by the school to pay that month's tuition. Having been at the hospital for almost the entire previous month I was a month behind so I was anxious to get there and get caught up. I stopped by the business manager's office and, after giving her the latest Ava update, I let her know I was there to make a payment. She smiled and said we were all caught up. I smiled and said no we weren't. Her smile got bigger and she said a very generous patron of the school heard Ava's story and took care of her tuition for the rest of the school year. I was speechless. "What the?" and "Who the?" were about all I could get out. She explained the person wished to remain anonymous so she couldn't tell me any more. I stammered a heartfelt "Thank you" and then an "I better go" when my eyes started to sweat.

DANCE MARATHON

Dance Marathon is the University of Iowa's largest student-run organization. The organization provides year-round support to pediatric cancer patients and their families. We first became familiar with Dance Marathon when Macy was a freshman at Iowa during the 2013-14 school year. She hit us up to donate toward the $500 she needed to raise in order to dance at their "Big Event." The Big Event happens in late winter each year. It's a twenty-four hour dance that celebrates the year's fundraising, provides activities for the pediatric oncology patients and their families, and commemorates the lives of children who have passed away from cancer. Participating students have to raise at least $500 throughout the year and then stay on their feet at the Big Event for twenty-four hours...with no caffeine! Macy invited Renae and I to attend the event to see what it was about. While there I couldn't believe the number of students that had given up their weekend to raise money for childhood cancer. It was refreshing and completely unexpected seeing a different side of the "me" generation.

That same year my son's high school (Alleman Catholic High School) hosted their first Dance Marathon and he became involved in the program. They raised over $14,000 that year. In 2014-2015, when he was a senior, he served on the school's Dance Marathon committee and they raised over $28,000. Over the next two years the enthusiastic and passionate students raised another $70,000 for Dance Marathon families. Not bad for a school of 450 kids.

In spite of our familiarity with Dance Marathon we really didn't know what they were all about. Obviously, we knew they raised money and we assumed it went into some big pot at the University of Iowa to put towards childhood cancer stuff. We didn't know exactly what that stuff was but, unfortunately, we were about to find out.

Had you asked me prior to August, 2016 to describe the typical college student, I would have used words like self-centered and apathetic. Today, I use words like selfless, loving, and compassionate. Though Dance Marathon has raised over $30 million in their 26 years of existence at the University of Iowa, we found out it is much more than just a fundraising organization. Way more. The Dance Marathon students made their presence known early and often in Ava's treatment and it wasn't long before we considered them part of her care team.

I believe every encounter with another person is the entrance exam into heaven, and students involved in Dance Marathon pass their exams with flying colors. Dance Marathon students stopped by Ava's room all the time to see if she wanted to hang out, even though she almost never felt like it. They usually ended up entertaining Renae and I instead. As accommodating as the hospital rooms are, being stuck in them day after day got painfully monotonous. It was always a joy, and a refreshing break, to spend time talking with them. Each week we were in the hospital they would offer us gift cards to local restaurants so we didn't always have to eat hospital food. They covered the cost of every one of our prescription co-pays during Ava's treatment. That was an immense help considering all of the medicines she was on. Throughout the year they sponsor free events for families of children that have received or are receiving cancer treatment. These events range from a family day at a pumpkin patch to a day of fun at Adventureland, Iowa's largest amusement park. We took advantage of these events whenever Ava had the strength. It was nice to be able to go somewhere other than the hospital for a change.

Speaking of the hospital, Dance Marathon provided substantial funding for the 11th floor of the new University of Iowa Stead Family Children's Hospital, completed in April, 2017. That floor is aptly named the Dance Marathon Pediatric Cancer and Blood Disorders Center. All pediatric cancer outpatient clinic visits and hospital stays happen there. The facility is incredible and with the new private rooms (the rooms in the old hospital were not always private) Ava especially liked not having to walk by another family's bed to use the bathroom any more. Dance Marathon tailors their support according to the needs of each family. No matter what the need though, they were always there for us with enthusiastic and heartfelt smiles, and we deeply appreciated the charity they showed Ava and our family.

We really looked forward to the first Dance Marathon Big Event after Ava's treatment ended. She was finally feeling well enough to enjoy it. She even got up in front of the three thousand University of Iowa students in attendance and told her story. The Dance Marathon committee had asked several months earlier if we'd be interested in sharing Ava's journey. After all they had done for us we couldn't say no, but once we said yes Renae and I and Macy and Brady started nominating each other to be the designated speaker. As we were arguing, Ava interrupted and said, "It's my story so I should be the one to tell it." We were all shocked since Ava is probably the shyest kid you'd ever meet. During her eighteen months of treatment and dozens of visits to her oncologist she probably said five words to him, and three of those you couldn't even hear. But she insisted and we were more than happy to oblige. She did an incredible job. Though nervous, she spoke calmly and clearly and captivated the large audience. I think she opened quite a few eyes and hearts and tear ducts when she showed the string of Bravery Beads she earned.

For each of her procedures, hospitalizations, medicines, blood draws, chemos or other treatment-related events Ava would get a special Bravery Bead from the hospital. Her string had around 2,000 beads, and it reached all the way across the stage and then back again. I got a bit choked up when I saw eighteen long months of what she had endured condensed into one phenomenally long string. Seeing it made me so grateful we still had Ava with us in spite of all she had been through.

The Big Event is basically a twenty-four hour love-fest. It is the culmination of a year of raising the spirits of and funds for families in need. Fundraising includes everything from T-shirt sales to over two hundred and fifty students soliciting pledges to run the 26.2 mile Chicago Marathon. In true Dance Marathon style, each runner wore a temporary tattoo on their forearm listing the names of kids with cancer. They called them the Mile Motivators. There was one child for each of the miles, so when things got tough on the course, the runners could look down and remember who they were doing this for. It would remind them the pain they were enduring is nothing like what these kids go through, so suck it up and keep going.

The students spent the weekend celebrating the families that had suffered so much, and the families spent the weekend appreciating the students that had given so much to support them. It was also a great opportunity for us to meet other families that understood what we'd been through. I was incredibly impressed by the DJ of the event. For twenty-four straight years he had given up this weekend (and sleep!) to keep the students motivated and dancing twenty-four straight hours. I could tell he did this out of affection for the students and the families in attendance. I'm sure there's a dance floor in heaven, and I know one day he'll be DJ-ing it.

Towards the end of the Big Event everyone, student's and families alike, gathered in a circle and sang along to the song *Testify to Love* by Avalon. The beginning of the chorus beautifully summarizes the work of Dance Marathon...

For as long as I shall live,
I will testify to love.
I'll be a witness in the silences
When words are not enough.

Family Time

As most parents of kids in college know, once they leave home you spend a lot of time missing them. You lament the days of old when you got to see them all the time, not just when they have laundry or need money. An unexpected gift of Ava's illness was the family time we got to spend together. Though not under ideal circumstances, since Macy and Brady were both students at the University of Iowa we were blessed that they were able to attend nearly every one of Ava's appointments and able to visit her every day in the hospital. In fact, Macy was a volunteer in the hospital's burn unit so she was almost always close by. Her experiences in the hospital helped solidify her desire to work in one, and she has since graduated as a Doctor of Occupational Therapy from Creighton University. I can't imagine going through this with Brady being away at a different school. It would have been unbearable for him and for Ava. God's providence was at work again when Brady's experience with his little sister, as a computer science student at the University, and in his extensive volunteer work with the University's Dance Marathon program, inspired him to enroll in graduate school at the University of Notre Dame to develop his data analytics skills in hopes of discovering ways to predict and treat diseases. This incredibly trying experience helped shape both Macy and Brady's futures, and the value of being able to go through it as a family was immeasurable.

MAKE-A-WISH

Prior to Ava being sick, we used to occasionally put spare change into those clear Make-A-Wish coin collector bins, mostly because Ava wanted to watch the coins make their way through the colorful chutes. We never gave much thought as to what Make-A-Wish does or who the money helps. We didn't, that is, until they called and wanted to help us. We met with some local representatives who told Ava to wish big. She could do practically anything she wanted with very few restrictions (no new house, dang it!). All she had to do was come up with the idea and they would take care of the rest. Ava thought it would be awesome to visit her homeland in China. However, since she was still in treatment when she was making her choice and we had no idea how she would be doing in a week let alone in several months, we told her that even though Make-A-Wish would have gladly arranged for her to go there, she needed to stay a little closer to home. After much reflection, Ava decided she wanted to go to Universal Studios in Orlando, Florida. So, in June of 2018 we did.

I can sum up the experience in one word, WOW! Renae and I joke that we'll never be able to visit an amusement park again because we will always compare it to our Make-A-Wish trip and know that going as "normal" people will never come close. We should have guessed it was going to be a special trip based on the hotel we stayed in the night before our trip began.

We had dinner at the hotel when, much to our surprise, our meal was covered when we were randomly "paid forward." The payers left us a business card with a young girl's picture on it. The girl's name was Keira and, coincidentally, she had passed away from the same type of cancer Ava had, rhabdomyosarcoma. Her family wanted to carry on their daughter's memory by transforming their tragic loss into a force for good. I'll let Ava's post on Renae's Facebook page provide the details of the experience…

> My name is Ava. I too was diagnosed with a childhood cancer, the same kind Keira had (Rhabdomyosarcoma). I was at a hotel in Bolingbrook, Illinois eating dinner with my family and the waiter presented us with Keira's card with money to put towards our dinner. He said it was from 3 ladies that wanted to pay it forward. Thank you to those ladies and I am looking forward to paying it forward in Keira's name.

And pay it forward she did. At our hotel in Florida there was a family behind us in the cafeteria line with a child in a wheelchair. Ava decided that's who she wanted to help, so she gave the cashier money to cover their meal and asked her to give them Keira's card. We can only assume this gift of love we received is continuing to ripple throughout the world.

The next morning we were greeted by a limo to transport Lady Ava and her Entourage to Midway Airport in Chicago. Since we were a little ahead of schedule, the limo driver thought it would be a treat for us to visit the Lake Michigan shore and see the sun rising on the sleepy Chicago skyline. He was absolutely right! We've been to Chicago many times but have never seen the city look so peaceful and beautiful. The backdrop made for some great family photos.

Our plane ride on Southwest Airlines began with Ava getting to visit the cockpit and talk to the pilot before takeoff, followed with extra attention from the stewardesses, including a skillfully crafted crown constructed from bags of airline pretzels and plastic cocktail swords. A regal crown for a deserving princess.

The royal treatment did not end on the airplane. The next several days were filled with people going out of their way to make sure Ava's visit was one she would not forget. At Universal Studios Ava was a VIP (Very Important Princess!). Every ride we went to, when Ava flashed her badge we were taken directly to the front of the line and placed on the ride. We were incredibly uncomfortable with this at first. It was somewhere near 195 degrees outside as we were escorted past the poor souls who had been waiting what probably seemed an eternity in line, wallowing in their sweat and misery. I imagined it's what the line to hell's bathroom looks like. We tried subliminally pointing to our Make-A-Wish badges to let them know we were legit, but I'm sure the multitude couldn't see past the sweat cascading down their foreheads, burning into their weary eyes. After a while though, we started to be OK with it. First, because we were feeling absurdly hot too, even without standing in line, and second, we realized a few hours in a hot line was easy compared to the month's of torment Ava went through during her treatment. She had earned the right to be treated special for a little while.

The Wave

Several days prior to the 2017 Iowa Hawkeye football season Ava developed a fever and had to be admitted into the hospital once again. Admissions had become routine by that time but we were rather excited about the possibility of watching the inaugural game from the new Stead Family Children's Hospital 12th floor. We had been hearing it was going to be a fun day for the kids and the fans were going to do something special for them. Then, as luck would have it, Ava got better and the doctors sent us home the day before the game. We tried to convince them to keep her one more day as she might have the bird flu, mad cow disease, or cat scratch fever, but they would have none of it.

We were not able to watch the game on TV but did see news stories of the fans' special gift. Even though we didn't get to experience it first hand, we were touched so many people took a moment out of their day to wave to the families in the hospital. It was so simple yet so beautiful. We obviously were not the only ones touched by the moment. As is typical with acts of love, the action moved well beyond its intended target and produced much collateral joy. It was a tidal wave that left few unaffected.

Three weeks after the "best new tradition in college football" began, Ava once again developed a fever and was admitted into the hospital. Though she felt good, she had to stay over the weekend this time. I'm not going to lie, I wasn't too upset. We were going to finally get a chance to personally experience the Wave.

The Hawkeyes were playing 4th ranked Penn State that day. It was the first night game of the season and it was fascinating watching the area around Kinnick Stadium come to life from above. I finally had something else to watch besides episodes of *Spongebob Squarepants* and *Say Yes to the Dress*.

As game time approached we made the trip from Ava's room on the 11th floor up to the festivities on the 12th. The hospital really went out of their way to make this a special event for the kids.

They had snacks, games and activities and gave everyone glow sticks and a big foam hand to wave with. The joyful atmosphere really resonated with the families. It was something we all needed. The anticipation heightened as game time rolled around. We stepped up to the glass and watched the Hawkeyes and Nittany Lions do battle for the first quarter. The game was great and the view was spectacular. Then it was time.

It's no secret the world is filled with problems. There's a lot of darkness out there. Add to that a child battling cancer or another serious illness and the world can feel incredibly lonely. Then, 70,000 people turn to your family and wave, to let you know they're thinking of you and pulling for you. Suddenly the darkness is dispelled and the distance between you and them vanishes. For a moment, all is right in the world. For families like ours, where things had not been right for a very long time, this moment brought some much needed hope and joy.

Unbeknownst to us, ESPN was there that evening filming for a story about the Wave to be aired on their College Gameday pregame show the following weekend. It was so well done and hit so close to home that I've probably viewed it fifty times. Plus, Ava got a few seconds of screen time in it. She's the bald Chinese girl wearing a mask towards the beginning of the video.

Ava was so inspired by the Wave she spent an hour after the game sitting in her hospital room window waving to people in the street below. Her face lit up every time she caught someone's attention and they waved back.

So Many Other Ways

As soon as we returned home from Ava's initial two week stay in the hospital, she was ready to go back to school. To ease the transition and prepare her 4th grade classmates for what was and would be happening with Ava (as if we really knew!), Renae and I went to her school to speak to her class. The American Childhood Cancer Organization had provided us with several free books and resources to help us cope with our new life as a family with cancer, and we used those to help with our presentation. We kept it simple...we explained that doctors discovered Ava had cancer, which means there are some cells in her body that keep multiplying even though they are not supposed to. To treat this, she has to have chemotherapy, which is a big word that just means she has to take very strong medicine to stop those cells from growing. However, because the medicine is so strong, it can cause Ava not to feel well and to lose her hair...so don't be surprised when she comes to school one day with no hair! We went on to let them know that she will probably miss a lot of days of school because she is either in the hospital or at home not feeling well. We encouraged them to keep in touch with her since she would miss being with them every day. The hospital also gave us another awesome resource, which was a big hit with Ava and her classmates. An organization called Monkey In My Chair provided a big stuffed monkey to put in Ava's chair whenever she was not in class. The monkey helped remind the kids that even though Ava was not there, she was still part of the class. We told Ava's classmates they could choose a name for the monkey, and eventually they voted to name him Bob. The students took Bob everywhere they went, even to gym class. Bob also came with a backpack, and students throughout the school would often fill it with encouraging notes for Ava. Those notes brought Ava and our family many needed smiles.

After being bald for quite some time, Ava wanted to see what it would be like having hair again so she asked if she could get a wig.

We found a wonderful organization called Children With Hair Loss that provides wigs at no cost to kids with medically-related hair loss. We requested a wig and it arrived just in time for her to wear it to the daddy-daughter dance sponsored by our local park board. It helped her feel like a normal kid as we were out there burning up the dance floor. At least as normal as she could feel with a partner who dances like he's being attacked by a swarm of bees. We had a wonderful time and I was so grateful to spend the evening dancing with her.

A couple of weeks before Ava's radiation regimen began, she had to have what the doctors called a mask created to hold her body in place while some of her larger cancer locations were being assaulted with radiation. It wasn't so much a mask as it was a hard plastic mesh bodysuit, since it covered the upper third of her body. As she lay on the table the mask would be placed over her and then clamped down, preventing her from moving and having parts of her irradiated that shouldn't be.

At our initial pre-radiation meeting when the radiology staff created Ava's mask, they informed her that the mask could be decorated any way she would like. A local artist donates their time and talent transforming the plain white masks into something special. We were told kids often have theirs painted to look like their favorite cartoon character or superhero. Ava simply wanted hers to be her favorite color, rainbow. Renae and I felt a little sorry for the artist since Ava didn't give any other details, just rainbow.

When we showed up to begin radiation Ava got to view her work of art. It was amazing! I expected nothing more than a rainbow painted across the chest. Instead, the mask was painted to make Ava look like a new superhero. I called her the Rainbow Warrior. The mask was covered in rainbow colors, complete with rainbow wings on each side of her head and a rainbow cape. It was unbelievably cool. Ava loved it so much, after her radiation series finished she took the mask to school and showed it to her whole class.

Ava received so many other surprise gifts during her treatment. People we didn't know would send hats and blankets they made along with very nice cards, prayers and well-wishes. A motorcycle club pulled up to the hospital one day with trailers full of toys for the kids in the hospital. Ava got to go down and pick whatever she wanted. A Harlem Globetrotter once visited her and taught her how to spin a basketball on her finger. She thought that was awesome and she couldn't believe someone could be that tall. On May the 4th (May the fourth be with you!), a local Star Wars costume club donned their authentic costumes and light sabers and invited all the kids in the hospital to the 12th floor to meet and interact with their favorite characters. Ava thoroughly enjoyed getting her picture taken with all of her favorite "bad guys." I thought the club's motto was quite appropriate..."Bad guys doing good."

During the Christmas season it felt like Christmas every day at the hospital. We received gift cards from a couple of families whose children had previously been patients at the hospital, including notes of support understanding what we were going through. Practically every day someone would knock on Ava's door with gifts from various generous souls. Santa had a lot of helpers in the hospital.

Another source of generous self-donation were those that donated the blood and platelets for Ava's transfusions. She received over a gallon during her eighteen months, all from people who probably had no idea what it would be used for. Their "blind" gift helped me see what an act of grace blood donation really is.

A Few Lessons

Suffering is present in the world in order to release love.
—St. Pope John Paul II

It's almost stereotypical to say God gives hope in unexpected ways, but I can't explain it any other way. Ava was diagnosed with cancer in 2016, which also happened to be a great year for Chicago Cubs fans. Having been a fan my entire life, and being used to saying "Just wait 'til next year," the 2016 season was nothing short of miraculous. Though we spent a lot of time at the hospital in Iowa City, we were able to mentally escape whenever our beloved Cubs played on TV. During those games we could take a break from our worries and whatifs and just be a regular family enjoying our favorite team having a great season. Each game was a short but sweet brain vacation—a family "braication."

I remember sitting with Ava in her hospital bed, celebrating as we watched Cubs first baseman Anthony Rizzo catch the last out of World Series game 7, making them world champions. After 108 years the wait was finally over! A dear friend of mine passed away when he was 94 years old and never got to witness his dream come true. It was certainly nothing I ever imagined happening in my lifetime. In the midst of my utter joy and disbelief I was overcome with a sense of hope…if the Cubs could win the World Series, then maybe, just maybe my little girl could beat this cancer.

At the beginning of Ava's treatment I had every intention of keeping a daily journal to track our experience. I think in the back of my mind I wanted something to hold onto in case things didn't end as we hoped. But, reality and exhaustion set in and I ended up writing very little. On August 10, 2016, a week after we arrived in Iowa City, I wrote seven short words, "When despair knocks, I let hope answer." This became our family's creed out of necessity. When suffering enters, especially the suffering of your child, desperation comes easy. The sum of all that could go wrong condenses into one massive weight and begins to crush you. After the initial whirlwind, Renae and I intentionally avoided reading about rhabdomyosarcoma. We had read enough to know that a good outcome was not in our favor, and continuing to research it would only provide ammo for the desperation we were trying to avoid. We decided to leave those worries to very capable doctors operating under the guidance of the Divine Physician.

People often asked how we could get through something like this, and our answer was always the same, "One day at a time." We learned that today is a great gift and putting too much energy into tomorrow wouldn't leave enough for us to enjoy the gift of Ava being with us right now. Dwelling on all that could happen would be debilitating. The scripture passage from the book of Matthew, chapter 6 verse 34 often came to mind, "So do not worry about tomorrow; for tomorrow will care for itself. Each day has enough trouble of its own." So, we chose to hope, one day at a time. Being bombarded with love from so many people provided fuel for that hope.

I was surprised how this experience made me aware of the suffering all around me. Not so much in a sad way, but in an epiphany sort of way. Being in the hospital so much we saw multitudes of suffering people. Not just patients, but their families and friends as well. So much suffering but, also, so much love aimed at the suffering, like a firehose to flames. Family, friends, and hospital staff caring for those in need. Few places have more compassion on display than a hospital. Then there were times I would be somewhere in public, a bit weary from all that was going on, and I would think to myself that no one here knows I have a young daughter at home with stage IV cancer. And it opened my eyes that I didn't know their stories either. Who knows what tragic situation the person next to me just came from. What circumstances they may be in the middle of that are turning their world upside down. What cross they are carrying on their shoulder as they walk by me. Though our lives are incredibly different, one thing we all share is the carrying of a cross. Though they are different sizes at different times, we all have them. And by helping another carry theirs, through some sort of law of spiritual physics, that seems to make the one we are carrying a little lighter.

In addition to learning to live one day at a time, we also learned to find the good in each day. Some days, the fact that they were offering General Tso's chicken in the hospital cafeteria was the day's highlight (I really liked their General Tso's chicken!). Honestly though, even on the bad days, just having Ava with us made them good days. One day, several months after treatment ended and Ava had become herself again, I was mad at her for something and raised my voice in a very perturbed-dad-like way. As I was doing this, I caught myself thanking God. I thanked Him that Ava was still here and I had the opportunity to be upset with her, and that she was active and acting like a kid her age. I was so grateful, but of course I couldn't let her know that at the time.

People who knew of Ava's illness would rhetorically ask why God would allow something like cancer to happen to a child. Many people have wrestled with this, including me. I'm convinced it was God who guided me to a YouTube video a few months before Ava's diagnosis to prepare me to personally face this profound question. The short, simple video was by Bishop Robert Barron, founder of Word On Fire Catholic Ministries. He is well known for simplifying the intricacies of the spiritual life. When I first watched the video, I found it so thought provoking I actually bookmarked it on my computer and watched it several more times over the next few months. In this particular video, Bishop Barron was responding to a famous atheist who wanted nothing to do with a God that would allow bone cancer in children. Here's an excerpt from Bishop Barron's response:

> ...The single greatest rant against God's injustice ever recorded (is) not in an essay by an atheist old or new, it's rather found in the pages of the Bible. I'm talking, of course, about the book of Job (pronounced Jobe). So we know the outline of the story well. Job, in one fell swoop, has to endure every type of suffering. So in one moment he is stripped of his health, of his wealth, of his livelihood, of his family. It's all taken away. And we know furthermore that Job is an innocent man. And so there he sits in agony from the suffering but also in a kind of theological agony. How could God have possibly allowed this to happen? And Job delivers himself in the course of that book of rants equal to those of (atheists) calling out God....Then in one of the most dramatic scenes in the Bible he calls God into the dock. "You know I'm innocent. Why am I suffering this way?" What ensues in chapters 38 and following is the longest speech of God anywhere in the Bible and one of the most dramatic speeches of God. What does he say to Job out of the desert

whirlwind? He says, "Job, where were you when I made the heavens and the earth? Where were you when I laid the foundations of the world? Where were you when I told the sea where to stop? Where were you when I stored up the wind and the hail?" He takes Job on a tour of the cosmos revealing to him all of the mysteries and anomalies including, by the way, a little introduction to two creatures, one called Behemoth, one called Leviathan. Probably a crocodile and a whale, creatures that Job probably never thought of. And God says, "I made them...I made them just as I made you." In other words, they're part of my creation too. Now what's the point? The point is, God is not so much answering the problem as he is situating the problem within ever wider frameworks of meaning. God is the lord of all of space and of all time. God has providential care for all of space and all of time. Whatever we're experiencing is in the context of this infinitely wider and more complex situation.

Here's a comparison now, with Job in mind. Take Tolkien's *Lord of the Rings*. You know two thousand pages or whatever it is. Imagine now one page of that book is ripped out and cast to the winds. Let's say it floats on the winds for months. It becomes further tattered. Only bits of it remain here and there. Someone now, who's never read Tolkien, stumbles upon this fragment of one page and reads maybe one paragraph of this great sprawling novel. Now maybe he picked up just a piece of bland narrative. Maybe it's a little happy incident. Or maybe he picks up Frodo and Sam in Mordor at the depth of their suffering and he reads this one paragraph and he goes, "Well, that's a terrible story. Whoever wrote that must be some kind of monster to have written that thing." That little fragment belongs in a page which belongs in a chapter which belongs in a sprawling two thousand page novel. We who've read the story know that that terrible suffering of Frodo and Sam is ingredient in ultimately this…great, joyful and life-affirming story. Here's the point. I'd say this as first response to (atheists). What do we see of God's providence? We see one tiny swath of space and time. One little fragment. One sliver of space and time. Do we see good things? Yeah. Do we see terrible suffering? Yeah. Both of them. (To say) this makes no sense, there's no justification, there's no meaning in any of it, you see how arrogant that is? How absolutely unwarranted it is. How can we possibly say, based on this little tiny experience of God's providence, that God's overall Providence has no purpose or meaning?…If you believe in God, and remember the premise for (the) question was that God really does exist… if you accept that God exists, you accept that there's a life beyond this one. That this life is not the ultimate horizon of existence, there's a life beyond this one. Once you know that, can you say, yeah, that the suffering of a child in this world, it's terrible. Of course it is. Bone cancer in children, of course it's terrible. But, is it nothing but terrible? Is it irredeemably terrible? Is it terrible, period? Or, is it perhaps ingredient in a much larger story? Is it perhaps even a route of access to a deeper and richer life?

As Bishop Barron mentions, this did not really answer the question, "Why?" But what it did for me was place Ava's illness as a paragraph, albeit a painful paragraph, in a much larger and unfinished, actually never ending, story. A story that includes countless people that showed us love in myriad ways. The bishop concluded with:

> The day on which Jesus was betrayed, denied, abandoned, scourged, unjustly condemned, led to his crucifixion, and left to die on a terrible instrument torture, we Christians call Good Friday. How in the world could you call that day good? Because that day is not the final day. That's not the ultimate word but beyond that there lies resurrection. To believe in God is to believe in that possibility, and that provides another framework for this question. To understand why Christians call that day Good Friday is the ultimate answer to Job and the ultimate answer to (the atheist).

One of the first things Ava asked after we found out she was in remission was when the next Iowa Hawkeye football game would be. She couldn't wait to be in the stands at Kinnick Stadium to give a supportive wave to all of the kids still in the hospital. You better believe we were at the first game of the 2018 season, waving our hearts out to the families going through what we knew all too well. The photo on the cover of this book was taken that emotional day. That game, or better said, that wave, marked the close of a difficult chapter in our family's life. One filled with fear, anxiety, and despair, but even more so with faith, hope, and love.

Though the Wave itself was not an integral part of Ava's healing, it is a great symbol of what was…people giving of themselves and loving us. The Wave is an act of love on a grand scale that mirrored the generosity we received daily by so many different people, from hospital staff and family members to coworkers, friends, and complete strangers. I'd like to encourage people to "wave" as often as possible, to as many people as possible. Wave with a smile, a prayer, a gift, a shoulder, an email, a Slurpee or one of thousands of other possible ways. And waves are not only for people with seriously ill children, for everyone this side of heaven is carrying a cross of some kind.

Epilogue

No one has ever become poor by giving.
—Anne Frank

Unsure of what to have for dinner on the warm and sunny early evening of Friday, August 9, 2019, we drove around town hoping we could decide what sounded good to eat. In the midst of reciting a litany of local restaurants, Renae's phone rang. She answered and I could hear the voice on the other end say he was one of the pediatric oncologists at the University of Iowa. "I hate to have to call you but I knew you'd want to know as soon as possible. Ava's cancer has returned."

Earlier that spring, we noticed a small, pimple-like spot above Ava's left temple. Ava's hair struggled terribly to grow back, and in that particular area her hair was barely coming in at all. She had an enormous amount of radiation on that side since it is the side where her initial tumor originated, so we were not surprised. Because of its appearance, we thought maybe this spot was a renegade hair fighting to break through. We kept a close eye on it though, just like we kept a close eye on every other little mark, bump, bruise or anomaly Ava's body displayed. We knew the chance of Ava's cancer returning was quite high, so we remained vigilant.

On May 20th, Ava had her scheduled four month scans to confirm she was still in remission....or to reveal she was in remission no longer. As you can imagine, there are few things in the world more stressful than sitting around waiting to hear if your child's cancer has returned. I usually don't think about it until a week or so before the scans are to take place. Then, during this time, my mind tries to loudly remind me of the devastating information I could soon be receiving. It makes me think of a scene in the movie *A Beautiful Mind*, when the schizophrenic Dr. Nash is walking along and you see these people alongside yelling at him, only to find out they are not real people, just the voices in his head. It's in these anxious times I am especially grateful for my Catholic faith. The Mass, Eucharistic adoration, prayer…Jesus uses all of these to give my mind and heart peace and strength. I often wonder how people without faith can get through these types of situations. It has to be a crippling hopelessness. I pray I never find out.

This round of scans was particularly stressful. By this time the pimple above Ava's temple had evolved into a wider, reddish bump. We anticipated bad news from the scan results, but to our surprise nothing questionable showed up on the images. She was still in remission! Ava's oncologist did not seem very concerned about the spot, but told us to keep an eye on it and let him know if things change. Otherwise, he'd see us for her next scans in four months.

We were obviously relieved that no cancer appeared on the scans, but in the back of our minds we still worried about what the little mark was. Since it didn't appear to be cancer we thought maybe it was some sort of radiation induced dermatitis. By July however, the mark had grown a little more and started getting darker. We continued to be very concerned so we made a dermatology appointment in Iowa City in hopes of getting some answers. We weren't able to get Ava in to see a dermatologist until August 7th, but once we got there, she shared our concern and decided a biopsy was in order. She thought it might be basal cell carcinoma, probably a side effect of all the radiation Ava received.

This seemed plausible since, sadly, one of the risks of many methods used to treat cancer is the development of a different cancer.

We were told the results of the biopsy would not be available for a week or so, which is why we did not expect a call just two days later. I was not at all surprised the oncologist told us Ava had cancer again. I was completely surprised, though, when he told us what kind it was. Instead of the relatively easily treatable basal cell carcinoma, it was a recurrence of the very serious cancer she started with, rhabdomyosarcoma. It felt like the oxygen had left the car and Babe Ruth had hit me in the gut again with his bat. We agonized at the thought of Ava having to endure treatment once more and wondered if her body would even be up to it.

I mentioned, previously, we've always told Ava she was one in a million and, due to her type and variation of cancer, statistically she was. With this new diagnosis though, her statistical stature went interstellar. No oncologist we questioned, including a leading national rhabdomyosarcoma expert from the Mayo Clinic in Rochester, Minnesota, had ever seen the disease come back on a patient's skin. On very rare occasions will it appear initially on the skin, but to recur there, unheard of. Curiosity got the best of me so against my better judgment I tried to research what we were up against.

Unfortunately (but probably fortunately), there was little literature out there to even research. I think I remember running across a medical journal that mentioned a man in his 70's from the Middle East experiencing this, but that was hardly a comparable situation. Eventually I found a journal article from 2016 discussing a young woman who had an experience like Ava, what they refer to as a secondary "cutaneous metastasis of rhabdomyosarcoma". Though her specific situation was also much different from Ava's, the article did contain one interesting fact. Between 1966 and 2014 only fourteen cases of this happening were reported in the world, and of those, ten were in children.

God wasted no time sending me a message of hope, though. The day after the doctor called, I happened to stand next to someone in the store who was wearing a shirt with the words from Phillipians, 4:13, "I can do all things through Christ who strengthens me." I was pretty certain God sent down an Angel dressed in that shirt to give that message to me and my family. I smiled and thanked Him for the reminder.

We knew Ava had the small tumor above her temple, but now we had to find out if her cancer was lurking anywhere else. The week after speaking with the doctor Ava underwent PET and CT scans to let us know what we were facing. To our amazement and delight the cancer was not seen anywhere else! It was nice to have a win right off the bat. Ava's oncologist showed us the scans from when she was first diagnosed and compared them to the new ones. It was like night and day, literally. The scans from her initial diagnosis had bright spots all over, indicating all of the places in her body where cancer was found. The new scans were dark, save for two small spots. One was the tumor on her head and the other was showing us her slightly infected earlobe from her new double earring piercing.

Now knowing how much cancer we were dealing with, Ava's oncologist had the daunting task of figuring out how to treat it. Usually when a cancer presents itself, there is a specific treatment protocol that is followed based on type, amount, location, etc. Not this time. Ava's body was leading us through a forest without a trail, on an uncharted island. At night.

After much deliberation and consultation with other oncologists, it was decided that Ava would have surgery to remove the tumor first, then, when she healed, chemotherapy and radiation.

Surgery day was grueling. Not only was the tumor removed, but once removed doctors had to wait for it to be analyzed to make certain the tissue margins were "clean," meaning no cancer detected along the edge of the tissue. Otherwise, they'd have to keep cutting and removing tissue until the area was deemed cancer free.

Once they got the green light, confirming no cancer remained, the plastic surgeon came in and grafted skin from Ava's thigh onto the fresh opening so skin would grow over the new hole in her scalp. After her head was taken care of, another surgeon had to come and insert a port into her chest and g-tube into her stomach. At the end of it all, Ava was a sore and bloody mess. Like a seasoned veteran though, she treated it like just another day.

After staying overnight in the hospital for observation, we got to bring Ava home. We had a bit of a challenge awaiting us though. When Ava was first going through treatment we promised her a puppy once life was back to normal. It took quite a while to feel back to normal so the puppy didn't arrive until a few weeks before Ava's cancer came back. Once home, we were faced with a highly wounded daughter and a highly active puppy wanting to jump all over her. We knew we had to keep them apart for a while until Ava healed so we purchased a three feet high foldable fence to put in the living room to keep the dog confined but still let them see each other. The plan looked good on paper, but when deployed it failed terribly. The energizer puppy just whined and barked once we put her in the fenced area. She wanted to be a puppy, not a prisoner. A lightbulb flickered in my head and I soon realized my plan was actually a good one, just backwards. The last thing Ava felt like doing was getting off the couch, so I freed the puppy and imprisoned Ava. I moved the fence so it blocked the couch and coffee table from the peppy pup. We decorated the fence with a string of lights and I sat back telling myself what a genius I am.

After a couple of weeks Ava healed enough to begin radiation and chemotherapy. It feels wrong saying this, but this time around seemed like a cakewalk. I guess I should rephrase that… compared to the first time around, this time was much less taxing on Ava's body. Of course that's easy for me to say, I wasn't the one being cut, poisoned, and irradiated.

There were only three chemotherapy drugs instead of seven, and all infusions were in the outpatient clinic, once per week. No week-long stays in the hospital. Though radiation was again every day for five-and-a-half weeks, it only covered a relatively small field on the surface of her head, instead of multiple deep sites within her body. She often experienced stomach pain following chemo, but only once did she experience a fever and corresponding hospitalization.

The treatment plan was made up of ten three-week cycles. All three chemo drugs the first week, two the second week, and one the third week. Certainly much shorter than the eighteen months for her initial diagnosis. Eight and a half cycles in, however, Ava developed severe colitis (inflammation of the lining of the colon) and had to be hospitalized. At this point her oncologist suggested this was probably Ava's body telling us it has taken all the chemo it could handle and we should cease further treatment.

That was a conflicting moment. On the one hand we were glad she wasn't going to have to endure any more chemotherapy, but on the other hand we wondered if she had received enough to defeat her cancer. By the grace of God and the prayers of many, scans on June 8, 2020, revealed Ava was once again, and hopefully forever, considered in remission!

This time, as before, was filled with so many acts of love toward Ava and our family. Relatives, friends, coworkers, hospital staff, teachers, and strangers again gave of themselves to lift up and love Ava and our family. Much of the generosity shown was in ways similar to when she initially battled cancer, but there were many new ways as well. One in particular occurred in September, 2019 and, instead of involving a quest for a Slurpee, it involved a request for beer.

On ESPN's College GameDay program (the same program Ava's picture briefly appeared three years earlier as part of a story about the Wave), a young man from Iowa waved a poster he jokingly made asking for donations to help replenish his beer supply. What ensued from that request was a national outpouring of affection to Ava and her fellow patients at the Stead Family Children's Hospital.

To the surprise of Carson King, the mastermind behind the sign, people actually started donating to his beverage fund. Even more surprising to him though, donations kept coming. He soon realized his request was turning into something bigger than himself, so instead of selfishly keeping the money, he decided to donate it to the Children's Hospital. Once word got around about his generosity, it rippled throughout the country. People everywhere wanted to be a part of this simple, infectious act. In the end, what started as a thirsty guy with an open heart evolved into a national act of love, with three million dollars being donated by thousands of people to scores of suffering children. I am constantly amazed how God can take our simple, seemingly insignificant acts and elevate them to works of great love when our hearts are open to it.

Coincidentally, we happened to be at the hospital the day Mr. King presented his $3 million check, and he was kind enough to let Ava get her picture with him. I was glad I could thank him personally for his generosity and let him know how much I appreciated and admired what he had done. That encounter echoes one of the reasons I wrote this book—to give a heartfelt "Thank You" to the countless number of people, known and unknown, who have given so generously and selflessly to help us in our times of need. My family humbly and sincerely thanks you all and prays that God continues to bless you as you have blessed us!

A Final Note

*The strongest people are not those who show strength in front
of the world but those who fight and win battles that others
do not know anything about.*
—Jonathan Harnisch

In a way, this book covers the easy part of Ava's battle with cancer. A few months after her initial treatments ended, she started feeling anxious, depressed, had flashbacks, terrible nightmares, and trouble sleeping. Classic symptoms of posttraumatic stress disorder (PTSD). Thankfully, the oncology department at Stead Family Children's Hospital employs a wonderful psychologist to help children like Ava. She informed us that once treatment ends, it's not uncommon for these kids to have difficulties in response to the trauma they experienced being cancer patients. This is a new challenge we are slowly but steadfastly working through, again with the help and prayers of many.

Ava was at first hesitant to share the information about herself in this book. It is only with her permission that I do so. She decided that she would though because she wants, in her words, "to help people and inspire them to do good."

Resources

Not all of us can do great things. But we can do
small things with great love.
—St. Teresa of Calcutta

University of Iowa Stead Family Children's Hospital:
https://uichildrens.org

Adoration Chapel:
https://catholic-link.org/how-to-go-to-adoration-eucharist

The National Shrine of Our Lady of Good Help:
https://championshrine.org

The Rosary:
https://www.wordonfire.org/rosary/

Fr. Ted's Kids Mission in Kenya:
https://frtedskids.org

Corporal Works of Mercy:
http://www.usccb.org/beliefs-and-teachings/how-we-teach/
new-evangelization/jubilee-of-mercy/the-corporal-works-of-
mercy.cfm

Spiritual Works of Mercy:
http://www.usccb.org/beliefs-and-teachings/how-we-teach/new-evangelization/jubilee-of-mercy/the-spiritual-works-of-mercy.cfm

American Childhood Cancer Organization:
https://www.acco.org

Monkey in My Chair:
http://www.monkeyinmychair.org

Children With Hair Loss:
https://childrenwithhairloss.us

Make A Wish:
https://wish.org

Word on Fire Catholic Ministries:
https://www.wordonfire.org

Jeff Hoskins lives in Illinois but considers himself a common-law resident of Iowa. He worked for Iowa schools for over twenty years, had two children graduate from the University of Iowa, and has one who is a patient at the Stead Family Children's Hospital in Iowa City. With three great kids, two good dogs, one beautiful wife, and zero tattoos, he would never be mistaken for The World's Most Interesting Man. He does, however, consider himself the most blessed.

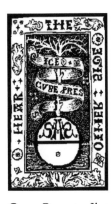
The Ice Cube Press began publishing in 1991 to focus on how to live with the natural world and to better understand how people can best live together in the communities they share and inhabit. Using the literary arts to explore life and experiences in the heartland of the United States we have been recognized by a number of well-known writers including: Bill Bradley, Gary Snyder, Gene Logsdon, Wes Jackson, Patricia Hampl, Greg Brown, Jim Harrison, Annie Dillard, Ken Burns, Roz Chast, Jane Hamilton, Daniel Menaker, Kathleen Norris, Janisse Ray, Craig Lesley, Alison Deming, Harriet Lerner, Richard Lynn Stegner, Richard Rhodes, Michael Pollan, David Abram, David Orr, and Barry Lopez. We've published a number of well-known authors including: Mary Swander, Jim Heynen, Mary Pipher, Bill Holm, Connie Mutel, John T. Price, Carol Bly, Marvin Bell, Debra Marquart, Ted Kooser, Stephanie Mills, Bill McKibben, Craig Lesley, Elizabeth McCracken, Derrick Jensen, Dean Bakopoulos, Rick Bass, Linda Hogan, Pam Houston, and Paul Gruchow. Check out Ice Cube Press books on our web site, join our email list, Facebook group, or follow us on Twitter. Visit booksellers, museum shops, or any place you can find good books and support our truly honest to goodness independent publishing projects and discover why we continue striving to "hear the other side."

Ice Cube Press, LLC (Est. 1991)
North Liberty, Iowa, Midwest, USA
Resting above the Silurian and Jordan aquifers
steve@icecubepress.com
Check us out on twitter and facebook
www.icecubepress.com

To Fenna Marie Semken
who inspires and cares
for those in need—
waving, cheering,
and helping.